# HOUSE CALLS

# HOUSE CALLS

Guidance on Common Medical Topics
From Your *Doctor-Next-Door*

Dr. Hollenbeck shares forty years of experience as a local physician
with tips on addressing illness and supporting high-level wellness,
including his personal journey of treatment and recovery.

## Terry Hollenbeck, MD

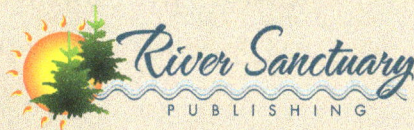

*River Sanctuary*
PUBLISHING

House Calls

Copyright © 2019 by Terry Hollenbeck MD

Book design by River Sanctuary Graphic Arts

Printed in the United States of America

ISBN 978-1-935914-89-1

Additional copies available from:
www.riversanctuarypublishing.com
Amazon.com

RIVER SANCTUARY PUBLISHING
P.O. Box 1561
Felton, CA 95018
www.riversanctuarypublishing.com
*Dedicated to the awakening of the New Earth*

## ACKNOWLEDGMENTS

My sincerest thanks go to:

- My wife Beth for her constant encouragement and her proof-reading of the articles to ensure that they would be understood by all who read them.

- All the wonderful patients over the years who allowed me to participate in their health care and helped me gain the knowledge, satisfaction, and experience found in this book.

- All the physicians and medical providers with whom I had the honor of working and sharing my practice.

- My local newspaper, the *Press-Banner*, for giving me the opportunity to reach out to the community with my articles these past ten years.

- Mary Andersen, who has worked tirelessly on creating and maintaining my blog: *valleydoctor.wordpress.com*, bringing my articles to many interested viewers from around the world. In the early days of my writing, Mary created a prototype book containing the first few years of my articles, giving me the idea to create this book.

- To Michael Wu, M.D., my local oncologist, and to Jeffrey Wolf, M.D., director of the multiple myeloma program at the University of California, San Francisco, both of whom have kept me going these past five years.

- Annie Elizabeth Porter and David Weiss of River Sanctuary Publishing in Felton, California, who so expertly crafted these articles into *House Calls*.

# CONTENTS

# Contents, cont.

# Contents, cont.

# Introduction

I used to go on house calls with my physician father when I was a young lad. I thoroughly enjoyed going into strangers' homes and watching my dad as he treated the homebound patient. House calls fell out of favor when physicians no longer had the time to do so, and also because of the modern changes occurring in the practice of medicine, such as the increasing need and use of X-rays, lab tests, EKGs, and other new technologies that were impractical to bring to a patient's home.

Be that as it may, as an urgent care physician for more than 35 years and seeing people in my clinic for their various illnesses, it dawned on me that a significant number of these patients had problems that could be simply diagnosed and treated without an actual office visit. Then I thought back to the old house call days when all this could be done in a patient's home. It made me think about what I would want to say and do if a patient was sitting in front of me in my office. What if they had a medical reference book at home that would do the same for them that I would do in my office? I like to think of this book as bringing my office experience and expertise into your home.

It occurred to me that the many health articles I have written for our local newspaper could be put into a health reference book format. The book, aptly titled *House Calls*, acts as my personal guidance to you, the patient. Through this book of my published articles, I thank you for letting me into your home to help you with your medical problem and to answer many of the questions you may have about your health.

## Food Allergies

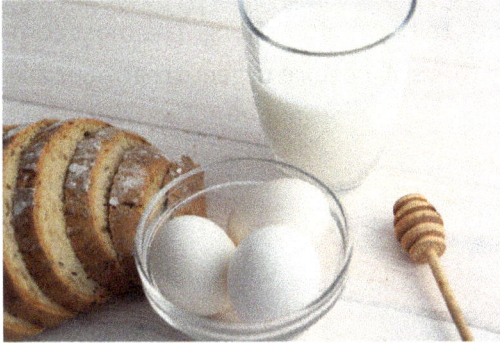

True food allergies affect about 2 percent of adults and about 6 percent of children. These reactions are triggered by the immune system causing symptoms that can be mild to life threatening. This is not to be confused with food intolerance, such as lactose intolerance, which is more bothersome than it is serious. An estimated 3 million children in the United States have food allergies with up to 200 deaths reported yearly. The impact of this disorder is felt at day care, school and camp settings, areas that are all integral to a child's life.

The most common allergies in childhood are milk, eggs, peanuts, tree nuts, wheat, and soy. Peanut allergy is of particular concern because of the frequency of true life-threatening reactions. Since the incidence of food allergies seems to be on the rise, it is increasingly important that everyone including families, friends, neighbors, schools, and restaurants better understand the significance of food allergies.

Risk factors for food allergies include family history and age, with allergies being most common in children. A child with one allergic parent has a 50% chance of having a food allergy, or a 75% chance if both parents have food allergies.

Some experts say that food allergies can be prevented in the first place, especially for at-risk children, by:

- Breast feeding, if possible, for at least the first 6 months of life

- Not offering solid food until age 6 months or older

- Avoiding cow's milk, wheat, eggs, peanuts, and fish until after the first year of life

Most food allergies improve with age, with the exceptions of allergies to nuts and shellfish, which can continue into late adulthood. Obviously, the best way to prevent a serious allergic reaction is to avoid the particular food. For many reasons, this is not always possible, especially because prepared food often has unknown ingredients in it.

Symptoms of a food allergy may occur within minutes to hours after eating. The most common, less serious symptoms of a true food allergy that still require urgent treatment are:

- Tingling in the mouth
- Itching and/or hives
- Swelling of lips, tongue or throat
- Wheezing
- Abdominal pain, nausea, vomiting

Symptoms of a more severe, life-threatening reaction needing immediate emergency treatment are:

- Extreme difficulty breathing or swallowing
- Dizziness, light headedness, or fainting

If you or someone with you is having serious difficulty with any of the above symptoms, call 911 immediately and have an emergency/paramedic provider offer prompt life-saving treatment, which involves getting a shot of epinephrine (adrenaline) and transport to an emergency room.

Quite commonly, a doctor has prescribed to the allergic individual an "EpiPen," with which the allergic person can immediately self-inject a dose of epinephrine and thereby save their own life.

For the family of an allergic child, sending the child to day care, school, or even to a friend's birthday party can be risky. They must trust that others will be able and willing to help their child avoid contact with the problematic food. Notifying all the proper authorities and caregivers in your child's life of their allergies is imperative in helping to keep them risk free. It is important that the general population, and particularly those who care for children, be aware of and protective of the food allergic child.

# Seasonal Allergies

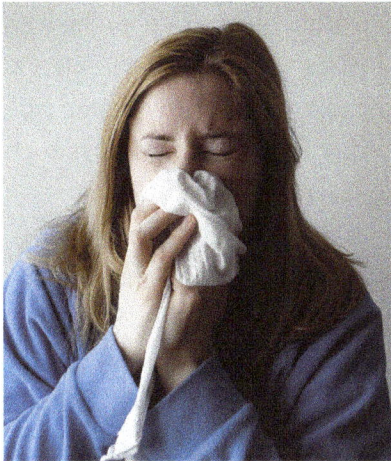

Seasonal allergies are commonly referred to as allergic rhinitis, a.k.a. "hay fever," if the nose is mostly affected, and allergic conjunctivitis if the eyes are involved.

Allergic rhinitis affects up to 40 percent of children and 10 to 30 percent of adults in the United States. It is referred to as "seasonal" if symptoms occur at particular times of the year or "perennial" if it occurs year round.

Common symptoms of seasonal allergies include sneezing, itchy eyes, nasal congestion, headache, and fatigue. These symptoms can have a tremendous negative impact on the quality of life and on productivity. American workers lose an estimated 6 million work days yearly to this disorder, as well as incurring costs of several billion dollars in medical care.

Seasonal allergies usually occur from spring to early fall, and are due to pollens from trees, grass and weeds. Interestingly, in this neck of the woods people associate the beautiful yellow-blooming acacia trees as the main source of allergies. However, the fact is that the acacia pollen is quite heavy and usually just falls to the ground. At the same time, birch, oak, and a number of grasses are the real allergy-producing culprits.

Perennial allergies, occurring throughout most of the year, are caused by indoor factors such as dust mites, animal dander, and mold.

Nasal stuffiness from allergic rhinitis can cause swelling and obstruction of the sinuses which can lead to a sinus infection.

There is a strong association between allergic rhinitis and asthma. Up to 50 percent of patients with asthma have allergic rhinitis. Sleep disorders in adults and a high proportion of ear infections in children are also associated with allergic rhinitis.

Treatment for people who think they have allergic rhinitis can begin with an over-the-counter antihistamine such as Benadryl or Chlortrimeton; however, they are often associated with the bothersome side effect of drowsiness. They should be avoided in children below 2 years of age and in the elderly. Newer oral antihistamines such as Claritin, Allegra, and Zyrtec, are now available without a prescription and cause significantly fewer side effects and are more conveniently dosed at once or twice a day. Steroid nasal sprays such as Nasacort and Flonase are very effective and are now sold over the counter.

Seasonal allergies can also affect the eyes, causing redness, tearing, itching, and swelling of the lids. This can be treated with cold compresses and with one of the newer oral antihistamines mentioned above. It would also be worth trying over-the-counter allergy eye drops, such as Zaditor, Alaway or Naphcon A. If these treatments aren't working sufficiently, see your doctor who can help you decide what treatment is best for your symptoms.

## Antibiotics

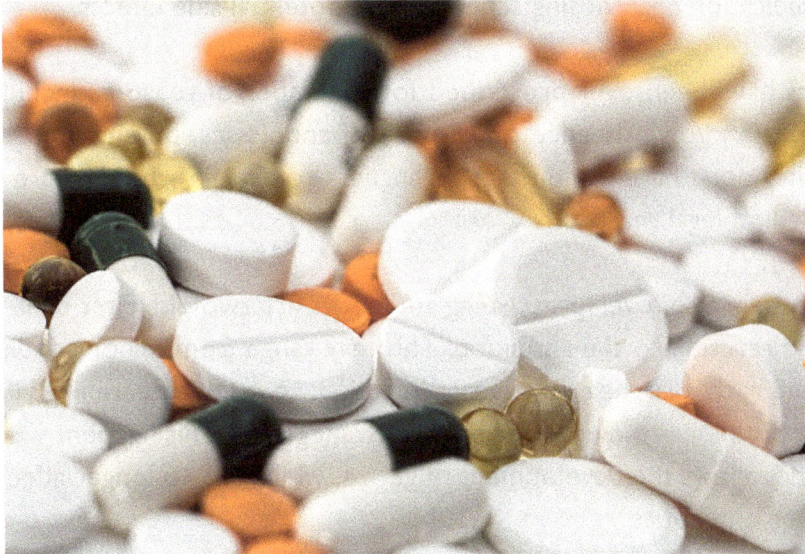

An antibiotic is a type of medication that kills bacteria or at least inhibits its growth, thus curing an infectious disease.

The first antibiotic to be discovered was penicillin, which was produced from a common mold and was discovered accidentally by Alexander Fleming in 1928. It wasn't used to treat disease until 1941 and became extremely helpful when it was found to cure the myriad of infections of the soldiers in WW II. Today there are more than 100 different antibiotics on the market, treating bacterial infections ranging from minor ones such as strep throat to life-threatening ones, such as meningitis.

As of yet, we have very few antibiotics that can treat virus infections. There are none to treat the common cold and only a few that can help treat influenza. However, bacterial infections, that cause such common diseases as strep throat, bladder infections, skin infections, and many ear infections, for example, can be cured by the use of antibiotics.

If an antibiotic is used, your physician will choose the one most likely to be effective against the type of germ causing your infection. Other factors in the choice of an antibiotic include medication cost, dosing schedule, and potential side effects.

Antibiotics have been over-prescribed for a number of reasons, including a patient's expectations and/or insistence on the use of antibiotics, physicians prescribing them because they don't have the time or willingness to explain why they are not necessary, and for medical legal reasons.

The consequences of over-prescribing antibiotics are twofold. First of all is the possibility of a bad reaction to the antibiotic. This may range from minor conditions such as a bothersome rash, diarrhea, or a yeast infection, to a life-threatening allergic reaction. The bigger problem is the emergence of resistant germs. This happens when the overuse of antibiotics allows the development of germs, which are no longer affected by most of the common antibiotics.

As opposed to the post World War II decades when drug companies were pumping out more new antibiotics faster than germs could become resistant, we are now in a situation where, for various reasons, drug companies are not putting in the resources to develop new antibiotics. This will become a serious crisis when we reach a time when many infections will not be treatable with existing antibiotics.

As I have emphasized previously, when seeing your physician for an illness, it is best not to have expectations of being treated with antibiotics. Rather, let your physician decide whether antibiotics are needed, and expect an explanation from him or her as to the reasoning behind that decision. You should also be given suggestions as to what you can do to make yourself feel better during the course of your illness while waiting for your condition to improve.

## Alcohol

The holiday season is a wonderful time for family gatherings and festive parties. The presence of alcoholic beverages is especially more prominent as we enjoy our eggnogs and toast in the New Year. Those who drink responsibly can appreciate the special holiday cheer while balancing it with good food and plenty of water. We've recently been told that alcohol in moderation may even have some health benefits especially for the heart. On the other hand, too much alcohol increases the risk of health problems and could damage your heart. It is associated with some 100,000 deaths yearly from injury and disease, with most alcohol-related deaths occurring in the young. Alcohol has also been found to be the direct cause of at least seven different forms of cancer.

A "drink" is defined as a glass of wine (4-5 oz.), a bottle of beer (12 oz.), or a shot of liquor (1.5 oz). Most people are surprised to learn that all these drinks contain an equal amount of alcohol. Or to put it another way, the amount of alcohol in one standard bottle of wine equals one six-pack of light beer and 2/3 pint of hard liquor. Moderate intake is no more than one drink per day for women or two drinks for men, and even less for those over 65. Of those who drink, up to two-thirds of women and one half of men admit to exceeding that amount.

Many people find it hard to admit they have an alcohol problem. Much self-denial is involved. Often those around a heavy drinker see the problem before the individual does. How can one tell if they are having a problem with alcohol? The following are a few characteristics of someone who may be on the road to alcoholism:

- Thinking about drinking all the time

- Trying to, but unable to quit

- Drinking more than you planned such as thinking of having one or two drinks with dinner, then continuing to drink all night

What causes alcoholism? No one knows for sure. A family history of alcohol abuse is common. Men are more likely to be alcoholics than women. Alcohol is often used to "self medicate" in an attempt to alleviate anxiety, stress, depression, loneliness, and anger. For those who think that alcohol will help them to sleep better, quite the opposite is true. One may fall asleep easier but have a difficult time staying asleep.

Excessive alcohol use is related to many health problems, such as liver damage (cirrhosis), higher risk of certain cancers, high blood pressure, high cholesterol, and increased abdominal fat, which puts the heart at increased risk. Other effects of alcohol include stomach pain due to bleeding ulcer or to severe irritation (gastritis). Psychological effects of heavy drinking include depression, anxiety, insomnia, and sexual dysfunction. Alcohol may have adverse effects on a baby during pregnancy, such as fetal alcohol syndrome and birth defects.

Alcohol also affects medication. Severe depression can occur from alcohol's effect on narcotic pain medication and tranquilizers. It can also increase the effects of sleeping medication. Alcohol can inhibit the action of Coumadin, a commonly taken blood thinner, and when consumed with an antibiotic called Flagyl, can cause a very unpleasant physical reaction. Patients often ask if they can drink alcohol while taking other antibiotics. I know that those who drink regularly will do so no matter what medication they are taking. The literature says that alcohol may lessen the effect of the antibiotic and may increase its side effects. My advice is to stop drinking while taking an antibiotic. If you choose to continue drinking while taking any medication, do so in moderation, knowing that there are potential negative effects. Talk with your doctor about the use of alcohol and medication.

Suggestions to help moderate your alcohol consumption if you choose to drink are:

- Pay attention to how much you pour

- Do not binge. Drinking less or not at all during the week, then having as many drinks as you want during the weekend, may cause significant health problems.

- Most importantly: If you choose to drink, DO NOT DRINK AND DRIVE. Always have a designated driver.

The bottom line is that if you choose to drink, do so in moderation.

# Cigarette Smoking

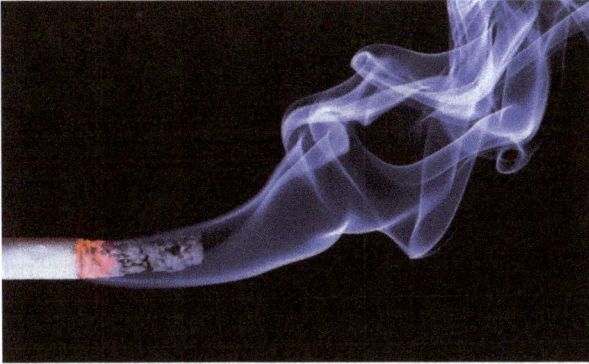

Good news has just come from the California Department of Public Health which has recently reported that the state's adult smoking rate has hit a record low. In 1984, 26 percent of our state's adults smoked. By comparison, recently, some 14 percent of the state's adults smoked. This is a very encouraging trend.

Tobacco use causes greatly increased risk of death. More deaths are caused by tobacco use (mostly in the form of cigarette smoking), than by all deaths from HIV infection, illegal drug use, alcohol use, motor vehicle injuries, suicide, and murders combined.

Cigarette smoking causes one out of five deaths in the U.S. each year with approximately 400,000 deaths from direct smoking and 50,000 deaths from indirect smoke. On average, adults who smoke die 14 years sooner than non smokers. Between the years 1960 and 1990, deaths from lung cancer in women increased more than 500%.

Smoking damages nearly every organ in the human body. Here are some of the more common health problems caused by tobacco products:

- Cancer of the lung. (over 20 times higher rate than among non smokers)
- Cancers of the bladder, mouth, throat, vocal cords, esophagus, cervix, kidney, pancreas, stomach, and certain forms of leukemia
- Coronary heart disease, which usually leads to heart attacks
- Double the risk of a stroke
- Blockage of blood flow to legs and feet, sometime leading to amputation
- Ten times the chances of dying from emphysema, a condition where lung tissue is slowly destroyed by smoke

- Reproductive problems such as infertility, early birth, stillbirth, and impotency
- Decreased bone density in the elderly leading to increased chance of fractures

It is estimated that more than 370 billion cigarettes are consumed by American smokers per year. Cigarette manufacturers spend  billions of dollars on advertising to lure people into smoking. What is the cost to our financially precarious health care system? It is estimated that cigarette smoking costs more than $100 billion yearly in health care expenditures and an equal amount in lost productivity.

I personally find all of this data shocking. We, in this society, must take a firmer stand against the use of all tobacco products. Every day, more than 1,000 American teenagers begin smoking. We need to do a better job of preventing our youth from beginning to smoke and getting those, young and old, who are already addicted to tobacco to quit.

For those of you who wish to quit but have been unable to do so on your own, your doctor has various treatment options that could help you.

# E-Cigarettes

E-cigs, also called vape pens or e-hookahs, are made to resemble cigarettes. They are battery operated, which allows conversion of liquid nicotine into a vapor that enters the lungs and is easily absorbed into the blood stream. There's no tobacco, flame, smoke, tar, or carbon monoxide, which is probably the only good thing that can be said for this product.

I'd like to touch upon some of the questions and concerns regarding electronic cigarettes:

*Are e-cigarettes safer than regular cigarettes?*

E-cigs have been promoted as a healthier, cleaner, and cheaper alternative to regular cigarettes. There's minimal research on the health effects and little data on long-term use. They are probably safer than cigarettes only because they lack the multitude of toxins in regular cigarettes. That being said, e-cigs are a nicotine delivery system, are highly addictive, and ultimately harmful because of the effects of nicotine, which is a potent stimulant drug that is probably unsafe for children, pregnant women and people with certain heart conditions. Newly released information describes e-cigs and damage to the gums and other tissue in the mouth as well as an increase in injuries from explosions causing flames, burns, and damage from flying debris. These products are not regulated by the FDA, and many are manufactured in China, a country not known for its quality control and safe products.

*Can e-cigarettes help break the habit of smoking regular cigarettes?*

There is no good scientific evidence that smoking e-cigs can effectively wean one off of regular cigarettes. In fact, one large study of 75,000 teen smokers found that those who were trying to quit smoking were less likely to succeed if they also smoked e-cigs, and many actually ended up smoking more real cigarettes. Better ways of breaking the smoking habit would be to use the strategies of behavioral counseling, nicotine replacement products, and prescription non-nicotine medication.

*Are kids smoking e-cigarettes?*

Since some 90 percent of long-term smokers began smoking under the age of 18, it's not hard to imagine the allure of e-cigarettes to our youth. The Center for Disease Control (CDC) has reported a disturbing trend that the use of e-cigs has recently more than doubled among U.S. middle and high school students. To make them more appealing to minors, manufacturers are making e-cigarettes in assorted eye-catching colors and candy flavors like watermelon, cotton candy, and bubble gum.

So with no proven health benefits and with too many questions concerning safety and long-term addiction, e-cigarettes should come with at least the same restrictions, warnings and health concerns as with regular tobacco cigarettes.

The bottom line is that for the sake of one's health, I would strongly discourage the use of any and all tobacco and nicotine products.

## Anemia

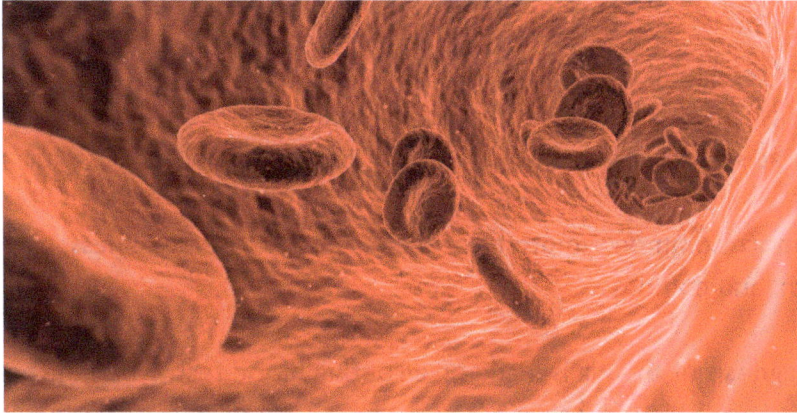

Anemia is a condition where blood lacks an adequate number of hemoglobin rich red blood cells, thus decreasing the amount of oxygen, which is so vital to the proper functioning of our bodily tissues. Within each red blood cell is a protein called hemoglobin, which is rich in iron and gives blood its red color. Hemoglobin is what enables red blood cells to carry oxygen from the lungs to all tissues of the body and carries carbon dioxide from the tissues back to the lungs.

Anemia is the most common of all blood conditions affecting some 3½ million Americans, especially women, children, and the chronically ill. It most commonly causes weakness and fatigue.

There are several main causes of anemia, one of which is due to blood loss, which can be slow and happen over a long period of time. Common causes of this would include problems with the gastrointestinal tract, such as colon and stomach cancer, ulcer disease, gastritis (inflammation of the stomach), and hemorrhoids. Heavy menstruation is another common cause. Rapid blood loss from surgery or injury can also cause anemia and usually necessitates immediate blood transfusion as a life saving measure.

Decreased or faulty production of red blood cells can also contribute to anemia. Some of these common conditions include certain vitamin and iron deficiencies, bone marrow diseases (often associated with some cancers), chronic kidney, and thyroid disease.

Destruction of red blood cells faster than the body can produce them also causes anemia. Such conditions can also be due to chronic liver and kidney disease, as well as inherited diseases such as sickle cell anemia and a blood disorder called Thalassemia.

Some of the more common symptoms of anemia are: fatigue, weakness, pale skin, shortness of breath, and dizziness.

Often, the diagnosis of anemia is made on a routine blood test, when the patient had no obvious symptoms. This can occur because the anemia develops over a very long time allowing the body to compensate for the lack of oxygen to its tissues.

Once the diagnosis is made, further  tests will be done to help determine the cause and best treatment for the anemia.

Anemia will be treated according to what has been determined to cause it. Iron supplements for iron deficiency anemia or folic acid and vitamin C supplements may be all that's necessary to cure some types of anemia. In other cases, curing the underlying disease will help to improve the anemia.

A blood transfusion may be necessary for more severe forms of anemia to rapidly increase the number of functioning red blood cells and help to more quickly alleviate the symptoms of the disease.

See your doctor if you have any of the above mentioned symptoms and expect a complete workup and proper treatment plan.

# Blood Clots

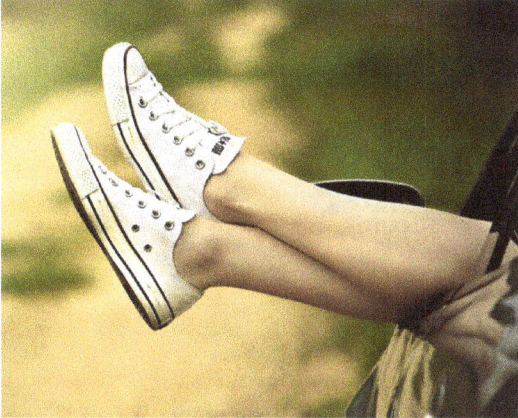

Many of us travel via commercial aircraft. It has long been known that with air travel, there is a risk of forming blood clots in the legs, a condition called deep vein thrombosis (DVT). Fortunately, this is not very common during travel, but there are other situations that place a patient at risk for DVT that I will also discuss. The major problem associated with DVT is that some, or the entire clot, may come loose and travel to the heart and then directly to the lung. This is called a pulmonary embolism and can be very serious and sometimes fatal. It is estimated that around 350,000 Americans a year are affected by DVT/pulmonary embolism.

There are certain factors that can make one more prone to this condition such as:

- Sitting for long periods of time such as when driving long distance in a vehicle or especially when traveling on an airplane
- Prolonged bed rest, such as during hospital stays or chronic illness at home
- Recent surgery or injury involving major broken bones
- Pregnancy
- Blood clotting disorder
- Cancer
- Prior history DVT
- Obesity
- Cigarette smoking

Symptoms of DVT are:

- Swelling of a leg (Usually only one is involved)
- Leg pain, usually in the calf
- Redness and/or warmth over the affected area of the leg

Symptoms of pulmonary embolism are:

- Unexplained shortness of breath and/or chest pain
- Feeling light headed or dizzy
- Coughing up blood

For most healthy adults, DVT is very rare. If you feel that you are at risk of DVT or trying to prevent a recurrent episode consider the following:

- Take precautions while traveling. Stay well hydrated with non alcoholic drinks. Take hourly breaks from sitting to walk around, or at least exercise your calf muscles while seated.
- Make healthy changes such as losing weight and stopping smoking.
- Follow the instructions from your doctor if you have recently had surgery or serious illnesses.

## Cancer Definition

Cancer is a group of diseases characterized by uncontrolled growth of abnormal cells that have the ability to spread and to destroy normal body tissue. Cancer cells may stay in one location only, or they can spread to all parts of the body by traveling through the blood stream or the lymph system. Once cancer cells arrive at their final destination, they begin to grow and destroy normal tissue. When cancer spreads in this manner it is referred to as metastasis, which makes the cancer more serious and difficult to treat.

Cancer can be caused by internal factors such as genetic mutations, immune system conditions, metabolic disorders, and also by external factors such as radiation or chemical exposures, tobacco or alcohol use, and even by infectious organisms.

Anyone can develop cancer. The risk of cancer increases with age, with the majority of cancers occurring in those above 55 years of age. Sadly, it can also affect the very young. The risk for getting cancer over the course of a lifetime is 1 in 2 for men and for women is one in three. In other words one half of all men and one third of all women, can expect to develop some form of cancer during their lifetimes.

Nearly half of all adult cancer deaths are from just four types of the disease—lung, colorectal, breast, and prostate. However, even with improvement of treatment options for many cancers, there has been very slow progress in successfully treating lung and pancreatic cancers.

About 15 million Americans are living with cancer. It is expected that over a million and a half new cases of cancer will occur per year. Almost 600,000 people will die each year from cancer, which works out to over 1,500 people a day. Cancer is the second leading cause of death in the U.S., exceeded only by heart disease. The cost of cancer is high with some 100 billion dollars being spent on direct medical care and treatment, and about 125 billion dollars of lost productivity due to premature death.

Common symptoms of cancer are:

- A change in weight, especially unintended weight loss
- Significant fatigue or unexplained increasing pain
- Changes of skin color, texture, or changes to an existing skin mole, or a sore that doesn't heal
- Persistent cough, difficulty swallowing, or hoarseness
- Changes in bowel or bladder habits

Risk factors for cancer include:

- Age: Since cancer can take a long time to develop, it most commonly occurs later in life
- Habits:  Smoking, excessive alcohol consumption, exposure to the sun, tanning facilities, and unsafe sex
- Environmental: Exposure to certain chemicals and second hand smoke
- Family history: Cancer development passed on through genes
- Excess weight and lack of exercise

There is some good news amongst all this information about cancer, and that is that the survival rate for most cancers is improving. This encouraging improvement is due to earlier diagnosis of many cancers, improvement of treatments, and an increasing awareness and importance of the various risk factors.

# Cancer Types

These are the most common cancers expected every year:

BREAST: Over 225,000 new cases of breast cancer among women and over 2,000 cases in men. Breast cancer is the most frequently diagnosed cancer in women. Increasing age is the most common risk factor. The survival rate has improved dramatically due to early detection and improving treatments.

PROSTATE: Close to 250,000 new cases of prostate cancer. It is the most common cancer for men. Increasing age is the most common risk factor. Fortunately, more than 90% of all prostate cancers are discovered before metastasis occurs, for which there is a 5 year survival rate close to 100%.

LUNG: Some 250,000 cases of lung cancer, which accounts for more deaths than any other cancer in both men and women. Cigarette smoking is by far the most common risk factor for lung cancer, and increases depending on the number of cigarettes smoked daily and the number of years of smoking. Death rates from use of cigarettes are dropping as a greater number of people are quitting smoking. Non-tobacco-related lung cancer is on the rise.

COLON & RECTUM: Over 150,000 cases of colorectal cancer. Fortunately, the rate is falling significantly as more people are having colonoscopies, which allows for the removal of precancerous polyps. Only 65% of eligible adults have been screened as recommended.

URINARY BLADDER: Some 75,000 cases of bladder cancer. It is found 4 times more frequently in men than in women. The most common symptom is blood in the urine.

UTERINE: (the uterus) Almost 50,000 cases. Early symptoms include vaginal bleeding or spotting, as well as pelvic pain. Obesity and exposure to the hormone estrogen are risk factors.

MELANOMA:  Close to 80,000 people will be diagnosed with melanoma, a potentially deadly skin cancer, which often metastasizes to other parts of the body. Major risk factors include family history of melanoma, the presence of numerous moles (more than 50), and exposure to ultraviolet rays mostly from sun exposure, but also from tanning booths.

KIDNEY:  Over 65,000 cases of kidney cancer. There are usually no symptoms early in the disease. Tobacco use is strong risk factor.

LYMPHOMA:  Close to 70,000 cases of lymphoma. This is a cancer of lymphocytes, a type of blood cell. Symptoms include swollen lymph glands, night sweats, weight loss, fatigue, and fever.

LEUKEMIA:  Around 50,000 cases of leukemia. Leukemia is a cancer of the bone marrow and blood cells. Leukemia is difficult to diagnose early because symptoms often mimic other less serious conditions.

PANCREAS:  Some 45,000 cases of pancreatic cancer. Unfortunately, there are very few symptoms early in the disease, and is therefore not detected until it has spread to other organs. By the time it is detected, treatment is often unsuccessful.

OVARY:  Over 22,000 women will be diagnosed with ovarian cancer. Symptoms are often nonspecific and include sensation of bloating, pelvic or abdominal pain, urinary urgency, and frequency. Diagnosis is usually confirmed by an ultrasound test.

CERVICAL:  (From the female cervix) Around 12,000 cases will occur in women. The most common symptom is abnormal vaginal bleeding. The Pap test is the most common screening method. The primary cause of cervical cancer is infection with the human papillomavirus transmitted by sexual intercourse. It can now be prevented by a vaccine, which is highly recommended for females and males from ages 9 to 26.

There are many other less common cancers. I have attempted here to highlight the most common ones.

# Cancer Treatment and Prevention

In previous articles, I described cancer in general terms and then discussed common cancers. Now I would like to describe various cancer treatments available and methods of cancer prevention.

There are a variety of treatments available today for treating cancer, including:

- Surgery:  This can remove the cancer or as much of it as possible.

- Radiation:  This uses x rays to kill cancer cells.

- Chemotherapy:  Uses potent drugs to kill the cancer cells.

- Stem cell transplant:  This is also commonly called bone marrow transplant. This uses stem cells which are found in the bone marrow, and are the precursors to all other blood cells. The cells are collected from the patient, or less commonly from a compatible donor, and then placed back into the patient after receiving a large dose of chemotherapy or radiation. This allows for the creation of a new healthy bone marrow and immune system.

- Hormone therapy:  Some cancers such as breast cancer and prostate cancer are worsened due to the effects of certain hormones in our bodies. Blocking these effects is the goal of hormone therapy.

- Targeted drug therapy:  This method allows an anti-cancer drug to specifically attack a cancer cell.

- Biological therapy:  Helps the immune system to better recognize and fight off cancer cells.

- Alternative medicine:  Not scientifically proven, yet found to be quite helpful for many patients. Such therapies include meditation, acupuncture, yoga, massage, and hypnosis.

- Vitamins and food supplements:  Also unproven but widely used with some success.

Although there is no way as of yet to prevent cancer, there are ways to reduce the risk of having cancer including:

- Stop smoking. Smoking has been associated with many types of cancer, not just lung cancer.

- Eat a healthy diet. Concentrate on fruits and vegetables and select whole grains and non-fatty proteins.

- Avoiding excessive sun exposure. Avoid mid-day sun, use sun screen liberally, and avoid tanning booths.

- Get plenty of exercise. At least 30 minutes of exercise daily is a good goal.

- Avoid obesity. Maintain a healthy weight.

- Drink alcohol in moderation if you choose to drink. One drink per day for women, two drinks per day for men.

- Schedule routine screening exams. Talk to your doctor about what exams you may need depending on your risk factors.

The bad news about cancer is that it is still so very prevalent in our society. As I have personally found out anyone can experience it. The good news is that through early detection and rapidly improving treatments, cancer patients have a much improved survival rate. Researchers are finding methods to mobilize our immune systems to better recognize cancer and to successfully overwhelm it in its early stages. Hopefully, we may be getting close to talking about cures for many cancers.

From my own personal experience with cancer and from many patients I have treated, my advice is that if something about your health just doesn't seem right, don't assume it's nothing to worry about. Listen to your body as only you can do. Don't take a chance. Being checked out by your doctor sooner rather than later could save your life.

# Breast Cancer

After skin cancer, breast cancer is the most common cancer in women in the U.S. Some 240,000 American women will be diagnosed each year with breast cancer. Although we usually associate breast cancer with women, it does rarely occur in men.

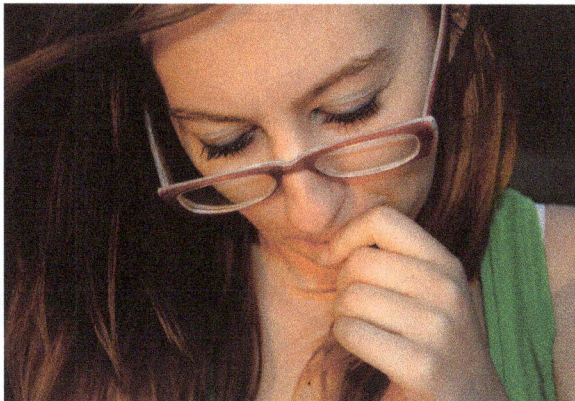

The most common symptoms of breast cancer are:

- A breast lump.
- Any change in the nipple especially discharge or bleeding.
- A change to the breast skin such as appearance of a dimple or pitting of the skin like the skin of an orange.
- A change in size or shape of the breast.

It is not clear why some women get breast cancer and some don't. It would seem that breast cancer is caused by an interaction between one's genetic make-up and/or one's environment. Some 10 percent of breast cancer can be linked to inherited defective genes passed down through generations of a family. Blood tests are available to determine who may have these genes.

Known risk factors for breast cancer are:

- Increasing age; more common in women over the age of 55.
- A family or personal history of breast cancer.
- Inherited genes.
- Beginning menstruation at a young age or beginning menopause at an older age.

- Post-menopausal hormone therapy using a combination of estrogen and progesterone.

- Drinking alcohol.

- Breast density

Tests and procedures to detect breast cancer include:

- Breast exam, including your own self-exams, as well as routine exams from your doctor.

- Mammograms.

- Breast ultrasounds.

- Needle biopsy (remove a specimen of the suspected tissue for examination).

- Women with very dense breasts should talk with their doctor about receiving more advanced imaging techniques.

Fortunately, the majority of breast changes do not turn out to be cancer. Even if you have had a recent normal mammogram, see your doctor if you find any changes in your breasts. Recent guidelines, especially regarding the significance of mammograms are changing, so also follow your doctor's advice about routine testing.

# Colon Cancer

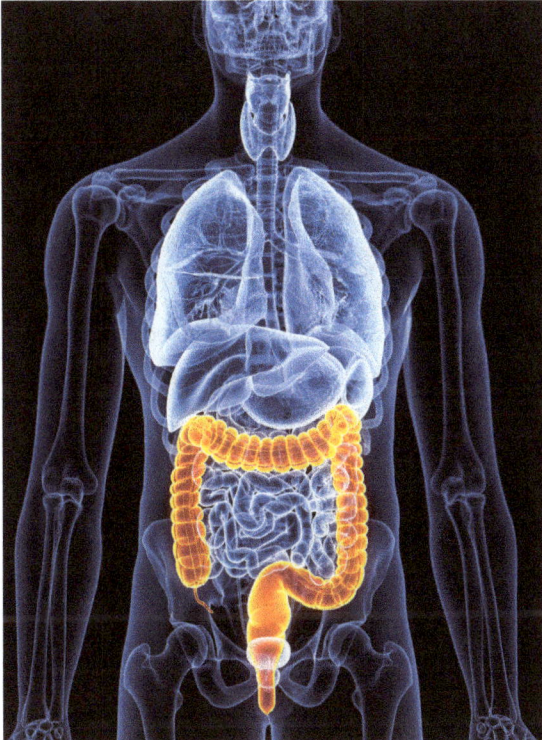

Cancer of the colon and rectum is the third leading cause of cancer in men and the fourth leading cause in women, and is more commonly seen in the western industrialized world.

Risk factors can include: age (50 years and older), family history of colon cancer, a high fat diet, smoking, and excessive alcohol intake. Most colon cancers begin from polyps in the colon which usually start out as benign, but after time can become malignant. Therefore, timely diagnosis and removal of the polyp can help to prevent the development of colon cancer, and thereby significantly decrease the mortality of this mostly preventative cancer.

A colonoscopy exam is the current best method for detecting colon polyps. During this procedure, the doctor can easily remove the polyp. Colonoscopy is essentially painless, is an outpatient procedure, and is a small price to pay for the possible early detection of colon cancer.

The more common symptoms of colon cancer include rectal bleeding and/or blood in the stool, a change in bowel habits, a feeling that your bowel doesn't empty completely, weakness or fatigue, and unexplained weight loss. Any of these symptoms should get you to see your doctor as soon as possible.

Your doctor will most likely do a rectal exam (don't be shy, as this is very important), perform a rapid chemical test of a sample of your stool to check for blood, take a blood sample to check for anemia, and most likely schedule a colonoscopy exam.

Surgery is the most common treatment for colon cancer. Chemotherapy and radiation are also often used depending on the extent and location of the cancer.

The bottom line is that colon cancer, if diagnosed early enough, has a very favorable prognosis.  If found too late after it has metastasized (spread) to other organs, it has a much poorer survival rate.

Talk to your doctor about colon cancer screening with colonoscopy, and check with your health insurer about what is covered. You should begin screening if you are 50 years old or older, or if you are younger and have a family history of colon cancer.

See your doctor if you have any of the above mentioned symptoms, and if you do, don't settle for anything less than a colonoscopy exam. Denial or delay can be a matter of life or death.

# Multiple Myeloma

Multiple myeloma is a cancer that causes an over-production of plasma cells, which are a type of white blood cell found in the bone marrow. Plasma cells function to produce antibodies, which are necessary for our immune system to fight infections. In multiple myeloma, the growth of the cancerous cells causes them to produce an over-accumulation of a certain protein called *immunoglobulin*, which travels throughout the body and can cause damage to various organs.

A common occurrence with multiple myeloma is that the plasma cells can enter normal healthy bone, causing osteoporosis as well as causing local areas of bone weakness, sometimes leading to bone fractures in the spine. Anemia is also a factor with multiple myeloma, because the plasma cells crowd out the red blood cells in the marrow.

The cause of multiple myeloma remains a mystery. However, there are some associated risk factors, such as:

- Being over age 65
- Being a male
- Being African-American
- Having a family member with multiple myeloma

Early stages of multiple myeloma may cause no symptoms. However, as the disease progresses, plasma cells accumulate in the bones and other tissues, causing these symptoms:

- Unexplainable persistent pain in any location of the body, especially the back
- Extreme weakness and fatigue
- Unintended weight loss
- Recurring infections

After seeing your doctor for any of these symptoms, you will have some blood tests done, and if there is some indication that you may have multiple myeloma, you will be referred to a doctor specializing in blood and cancer diseases. Further testing can prove or disprove whether or not one has multiple myeloma.

Therapeutic options include undergoing up to four months of chemotherapy, followed by a stem cell transplant.

What I have learned from my own experience (see my story "From Doctor to Cancer Patient" at the beginning of this book) is that it is important to recognize early symptoms and see your doctor about your concerns. As with any cancer, the sooner it is detected and treated, the better the chance of survival. If you or a loved one have any of the above mentioned risk factors and unexplainable symptoms, see your doctor.

Researchers are developing new treatments for cancer in general, and for multiple myeloma in particular. One of the new and exciting directions in cancer treatment involves the use of our own immune systems to fight the disease. Also, the rapidly expanding field of genetics also will play a big role in diagnosing and treating cancer.

For example, there is a new drug is called Daratumumab, or more commonly referred to as Darzalex. It is in a new class of drugs called monoclonal antibodies. The drug binds itself to a marker on the surface of the cancerous myeloma cell, directly affecting the cell as well as enabling the body's own immune cells to kill the myeloma cells. There is an ongoing search for new drugs because the chemo drugs for myeloma typically work for a period of time before losing effectiveness. Then a new and different treatment is undertaken.

Of course, those of us with cancer hope to survive long enough to benefit from the new treatments on the horizon. Hopefully in the near future as we develop a better understanding of cancer, it will, in many cases, become a mostly preventable and curable disease.

# Oral Cancer

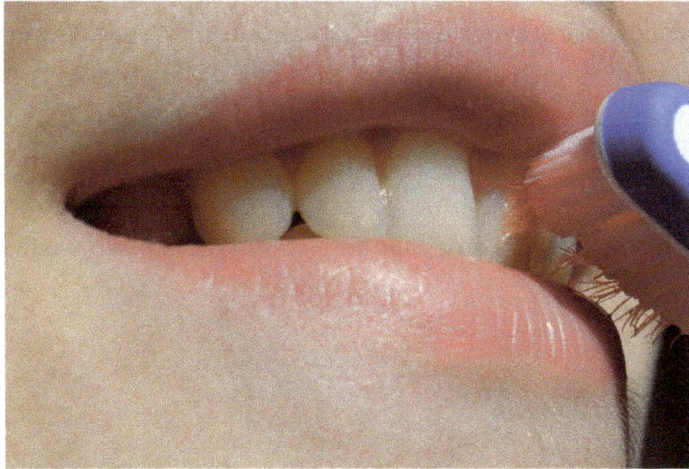

Each year, about 30,000 cases of newly diagnosed oral cancer will be found in the U.S., causing some 8,000 deaths. About 95 percent occur in people greater than 40 years of age. The average age at time of diagnosis is 60 years, and men are twice as likely to be diagnosed with oral cancer than women. When oral cancer is found early, patients have an 80 to 90 percent chance of survival. Most all tissues found within the mouth including the lining of the mouth, tongue, lips, gums, and roof of mouth can become cancerous.

Symptoms include:

- A sore or ulcer within the mouth that does not heal
- A white or red patch within the mouth
- A lump on the lip, mouth, or tongue
- Unusual pain, numbness, or bleeding in the mouth

Those with the highest risk of oral cancer are people who smoke or chew tobacco, drink heavy amounts of alcohol, or have a heavy exposure to the sexually transmitted human papillomavirus (HPV). In fact, the largest and fastest growing population of oral cancer patients are young non smokers with history of HPV.

Make sure that when you visit your dentist or hygienist, they do a thorough oral exam.

Talk with your child's primary care physician about HPV vaccination, which has a high probability of preventing such an infection, thus decreasing the odds of contracting HPV induced oral cancer.

Remember that if you have any of the previously mentioned symptoms, or if you have a sore throat or swallowing problems that persist more than two weeks, see your doctor.

# Ovarian Cancer

Each year in the United States, more than 22,000 women are diagnosed with ovarian cancer. It is referred to as the "silent killer" because it usually isn't found until it has spread to other areas of the body. Early detection is of utmost importance. Only about 20 percent of ovarian cancers are found before they spread beyond the ovaries. Women who are diagnosed in the earliest stages have a favorable survival rate, which is very encouraging.

Most common risk factors:

- Family history of ovarian cancer, especially in a mother or sister
- Family history of breast or colon cancer, or if you already have had either of these cancers
- Being a woman over age 50
- Never having had children
- Having taken certain fertility drugs
- Obesity
- Certain inherited breast cancer genes, although not common, have a high association with ovarian cancer when they are present

Most common symptoms:

- Abdominal fullness, pressure, bloating, or swelling
- Frequent urination
- Discomfort or pain in the pelvic region
- Persistent indigestion, nausea, or gas
- Unexplained change in bowel habit, especially constipation
- Unexplained sudden weight gain or loss

I can't emphasize enough the importance of seeing your doctor if you have bloating, pressure, or swelling of your abdomen or pelvis lasting more than a few weeks. If you've seen your doctor for these symptoms and have received a diagnosis other than ovarian cancer and your symptoms don't improve from the recommended treatment, then see your doctor again, or get a second opinion. Make sure that a pelvic exam is performed as well as an ultrasound exam if you and your doctor are suspicious of ovarian cancer.

Again, an early diagnosis of ovarian cancer will increase your odds of survival. You must not wait more than a few weeks to see your doctor if you have any of the above symptoms, and even more so if you also have any of the known risk factors. Expect your doctor to consider the possibility of ovarian cancer and to perform or order the appropriate tests.

# Prostate Cancer

Prostate cancer is one of the most common cancers affecting American men. Over one million men in the U.S. currently are living with the diagnosis of prostate cancer and many more men have it and are unaware of it. It is estimated to affect one out of six men in our population.

The majority of men with prostate cancer are in their 70's or 80's. Many of them are not aware of their cancer, and will likely die of other illnesses before they would ever succumb to prostate cancer.

The prostate gland is a walnut-shaped gland in men that is located between the bladder and the base of the penis, and produces fluid to help transport sperm. In many cases, the cancer is very slow growing, is confined to the gland itself, and may not spread for years or decades. Unfortunately, sometimes it can be more aggressive and spread rapidly. This is especially true when diagnosed in younger men. As with all cancers, the sooner it is detected, the better chance of a cure.

Prostate cancer usually doesn't produce noticeable symptoms in its early stages, so therefore many cases of prostate cancer aren't detected until found during a routine exam, or when it has spread.

When urinary signs and symptoms do occur they include:
- A less strong urine stream
- An intense urge to urinate
- Frequency of urination
- Blood in the urine
- Low abdominal pain

The main risk factors are:

- Older age. Rare before age 40, but increasing with every passing decade.

- More common in African-Americans

- Family history, especially in father or brother

- High fat diet

- Treatment with the male hormone testosterone

Men need to be screened for prostate cancer. One method of screening is the PSA blood test. I would advise that men follow the recommendations of the American Urological Society and have their first PSA test at age 40. If the result is low then with the advice of your doctor, the next test would be at age 45 and then once a year thereafter.

Of equal or even greater importance is the rectal exam. Although most men tend to shy away from this exam, it is extremely important in diagnosing prostate cancer and has saved many lives. The exam is slightly uncomfortable, but is quick and simple. The doctor will feel the surface of the prostate gland through the rectal wall, and will check the surface of the gland for any abnormalities such as bumps, hardness, and enlargement.

The bottom line is, men need to talk with their doctor about prostate screening by age 40. I understand the reluctance that many men may feel when they contemplate having this recommended yearly exam, but I can't emphasize enough the importance of routine prostate screening which can prolong and enhance a man's life.

# Skin Cancer

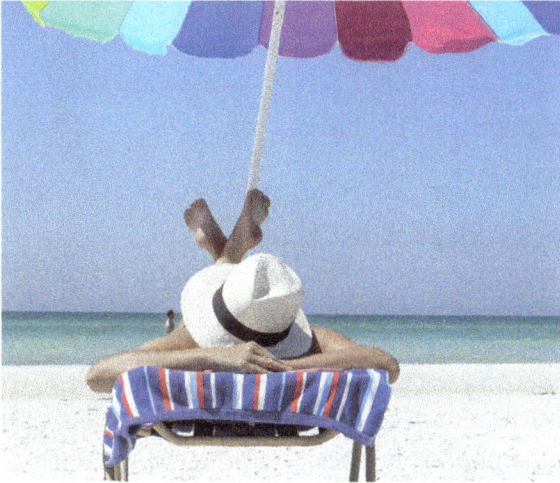

Skin cancer occurs when DNA changes cause the skin cells to form a cancerous growth. Most of the common skin cancers are caused by exposure to the sun and its ultraviolet light rays that damage the skin. Even one bad sun burn as a child can increase the chance of skin cancer in adulthood.

I would like to discuss the three most common types of skin cancer:

**Basal cell carcinoma** — The most common of skin cancers. Can appear as an open sore, a flesh colored or brown flat lesion, or as a waxy pearly bump. Usually not serious and treated by removal of the lesion.

**Squamous cell carcinoma** — Appears as a red small bump or a scaly, flat, crusty lesion. It is usually not serious, but can rarely be more aggressive. It also needs removal.

**Melanoma** — The least common of the three, but most potentially deadly. It is usually found on sun exposed areas of the skin, but can rarely be found in other parts of the body, such as the eyes, some internal organs, and under finger/toe nails. Melanoma often presents as a new, usually dark colored lesion or it can present as a change in an existing mole

If you have moles, remember the letters ABCDE to help identify the changes to melanoma:

- A is for asymmetry. If you draw a line through the lesion the halves will not match.
- B is for irregular shaped border.

- C is for change in color, usually becoming darker.
- D is for diameter (a mole becoming greater than 1/4 inch).
- E  is for evolving (changing).

Factors that may influence skin cancer are:

- A history of sunburns and excessive exposure to the sun.
- Fair skin and/or having blond or red hair.
- Moles and other common skin lesions such as actinic keratoses (non cancerous skin lesions).
- A family or personal history of skin cancer.

The most important thing to help prevent these common skin cancers is to avoid exposure to ultra violet light, whether naturally from the sun or artificially from tanning booths.

The bottom line is that if you or someone close to you sees something suspicious on your skin, even  your scalp with a full head of hair, see your doctor as soon as possible. Remember that the sooner a skin cancer is identified, the more successful will be the treatment, and potential cure.

## Childhood Fever

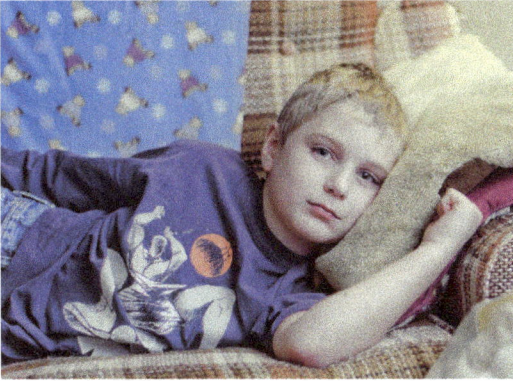

Fever is an elevation of body temperature and indicates that one is fighting off an infection. Fever is merely a symptom of an illness, and is often helpful in fighting the infection by activating cells of the immune system.

Some people may fear that a high fever can cause brain damage, but this would be very unlikely to happen. What may occur, is that a young child could suffer a seizure from a fever, but this is due more to how quickly a fever rises than how high the temperature really is. Although extremely frightening for all involved, such a seizure usually leaves no lasting problems for the child, but still needs urgent evaluation at your nearest emergency room.

Your child's temperature mostly needs treatment to make your child more comfortable. If your child has a mild fever but is active, playful, and eating well, the fever does not need to be treated. Treating the fever does not make the infection go away faster. Your child needs a medical evaluation if under 3 months of age, any child with a fever of 102 degrees or higher, is vomiting, or not responding normally.

Fever is usually treated with either acetaminophen (Tylenol) or ibuprofen (Advil, Motrin). These drugs come in various forms such as liquid, chewable, and tablet depending on the age of the child. Read the directions very carefully to give the proper dose. These drugs are quite safe when correct dosage is given. Do not use common kitchen spoons to measure doses. Instead use a measuring device such as a syringe, measuring cup, or measuring spoon specifically made for liquid medicines.

If a child with a fever is shivering keep them warm. When shivering stops, clothing and blankets can be removed to help the child cool down. Encourage plenty of liquids to drink.

The child may be cooled with lukewarm sponge baths which should be discontinued if shivering begins. Never use alcohol on the child's skin as this can be harmful.

If you are concerned about your child who has a fever and appears ill, see your doctor.

# Cold and Cough Treatment for Infants and Children

Every parent of a sick child wants to do whatever possible to make the child feel better. Most cold and flu like illnesses in children are caused by viruses, which will be cured by the child's own immune system. Many over the counter cold medications for children have been withdrawn for safety reasons. The Federal Drug Administration now warns against giving children younger than 4 years any over the counter medications other than pain and fever relievers.

Here are suggestions for symptomatic relief of your child's cold or flu like illness:

1.  Encourage the child to drink plenty of fluids to prevent dehydration and to help thin out mucous. Contrary to popular opinion milk has not been proven to increase mucous or to thicken it.

2.  Fever or pain can be controlled using either acetaminophen (Tylenol) or Ibuprofen (Advil), giving accurate and consistent doses every six hours.

3.  Saline irrigations:  for infants, use rubber bulb suction with saline (salt) nose drops to remove mucous. A saline nose spray can be used for older children. These products are available at your pharmacy.

4.  Use a cool mist humidifier or vaporizer in the child's room. To prevent contamination, the water should be replaced daily, and the machine cleansed regularly, according to the manufacturer's recommendations. Keep indoor relative humidity at about 40 percent to 50 percent.

5.  If a medication such as Tylenol or Advil is given, I do not advise the use of household silverware spoons for dose measurement. Teaspoons found in our kitchens can vary in size and should only be used for eating, not for measuring liquid medication. Proper measuring devices using units of milliliters usually come with the medicine or can be obtained from the pharmacist.

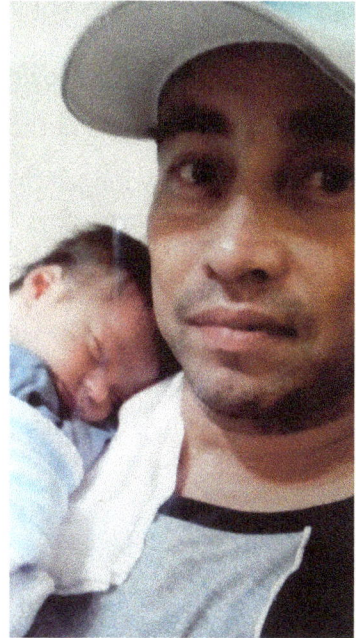

6.  Honey can relieve cough by increasing saliva, which coats the throat and relieves irritation. Suggested doses are, half a teaspoon for children between 1 to 5 years, 1 teaspoon for children 6 to 11 years, and 2 teaspoons for children 12 years and older. Do not give honey to a child younger than one year of age.

See your health care provider immediately for:

- A child under 3 months of age with any fever
- A child younger than 2 years with a fever that lasts longer than two to three days
- A child who complains of an earache or a severe sore throat
- A child who has thick green nasal discharge for more than one week
- Mild illness symptoms that are not improving in seven to ten days
- Any child who, in your opinion, seems very ill

Whether you have a newborn or a teenage child, what he/she eats is important to both physical and mental development. The following are recommendations supported by the American Academy of Pediatrics.

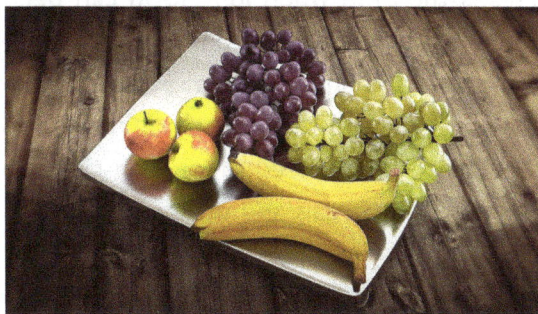

## Infants

From birth to 12 months, it's all about milk, whether it's breast milk, iron fortified formula, or a combination of the two. Whole milk is not to be given during this time. At four to six months, babies can begin solid foods such as iron fortified baby cereal, strained fruits, vegetables, and pureed meats. Fat restriction at this age is usually not necessary since fat helps to develop the brain and nerves.

## Preschoolers and Toddlers

At 12 months, children who have weaned off of breast feeding, may begin whole milk. Low fat milk would be better if there is a strong family history of obesity or heart disease. Calcium is necessary during this time to help build strong healthy bones and teeth. Milk is still one of the best calcium sources along with fortified cereals and juices. Fiber is also important to help fight obesity, promote digestion, and prevent constipation.

## Elementary School

Protein is important in this group, and if a child won't eat meat, then plenty of protein can be found in beans, eggs, nuts, and peanut butter. At this age kids will start eating more not-so-healthy snacks and fast foods. It is important to monitor their intake of fats, salt, and the ever increasing consumption of sugar in all its many forms.

## Teens

This is the time when junk food can become a bigger part of the diet. It's also when some kids become very conscious of their weight and may develop eating disorders, such as bulimia and anorexia. Calorie requirements increase, as does the need for calcium. Low fat milk and calcium-rich fortified foods are still very important. Girls who begin menstruating will need more iron rich foods such as meat, poultry, vegetables, beans, and fortified cereals and grains.

It is also now recommended that all children, beginning in the first two months of life, receive at least 400 IU of vitamin D daily. Discuss this with your doctor.

Getting our children to eat a healthy diet may not be an easy task. There's too much childhood obesity (1 in 3 children in America), as well as diabetes and even heart disease. We need to monitor our children's eating preferences and habits, and be diligent about encouraging and explaining to them the benefits of a healthy well balanced diet. For parents this may be a constant battle, but one well worth fighting to help ensure that our children will grow up to be healthy adults.

# Backpack Safety

I recall a time when my daughter my daughter was a youngster and she complained to me about her back pain. I wasn't sure what was causing her discomfort until one day when I had to lift her school back pack out of my car. I almost threw my own back out! I couldn't believe how heavy it was. It weighed 20 pounds and my daughter weighed 80 pounds!

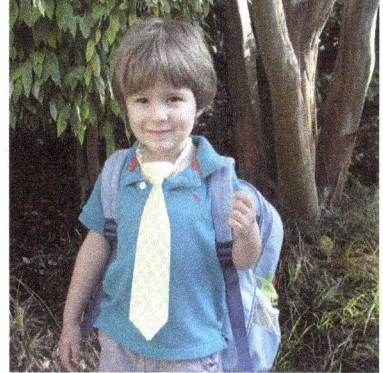

Carrying a heavy backpack can be a source of low level trauma leading to shoulder, neck, and back pain in children. This is especially true for those school kids in middle and high school, who have neither a locker nor desk to store their books during the school day.

Experts recommend that children carry backpacks that weigh 10 percent or less than their body weight and no more than 15 percent.

The way a backpack is carried may contribute to the problem. Some kids wear their backpack over only one shoulder often because it's "cool" or just plain easier. This causes them to walk unbalanced, thus causing abnormal stresses on their young developing spines.

A heavy backpack on a bicycle rider may make one top heavy and less stable on the bike, potentially leading to accidental injuries.

A good back pack should have the following features:
- Be lightweight
- Have two wide-padded shoulder straps
- A padded back, for comfort and injury protection
- A waist belt and multiple compartments to help distribute weight more evenly

The following are suggestions for kids who use backpacks:

- Pick up the bag properly by bending at the knees before lifting and using both hands.

- Keep straps tight for proper fit.

- Don't carry around unnecessary personal items.

- Use all of the backpack's compartments, putting the heavier items such as textbooks near the center of the back.

- Take advantage of using available online books that don't have to be carried around.

We, as parents, need to be aware of this potential problem, and be proactive in helping our children to make best use of their backpacks.

If your child continues to have back pain even after making the above adjustments, or has numbness, weakness or tingling in the arms or legs, consult with your doctor.

# Halloween Safety

Halloween is a time when many of our kids will be out trick or treating. It's an exciting night for all of the costumed children. To help ensure safety, I'll share some tips from the American Society of Pediatrics, as well as some of my own thoughts.

All Dressed Up:

- Costumes should be bright, reflective, flame resistant, and properly fitting.

- Consider facial make up and hats as an alternative to a face mask that can block vision.

- If a sword, cane, or stick is used, it should not be too sharp or too long.

On The Trick-Or-Treat Trail:

- A parent or responsible adult must accompany young children on their rounds in the neighborhood.

- Only go to well lit homes and do not enter the house.

- Remain on well lit streets and use sidewalk or far edge of the road facing traffic.

- Carry a flashlight and a cell phone.

- Cross the street at crosswalks and never cross between parked cars.

- Older children and teens going out without an adult, should let parents know where they are going, have a curfew to return, and stay in a group.

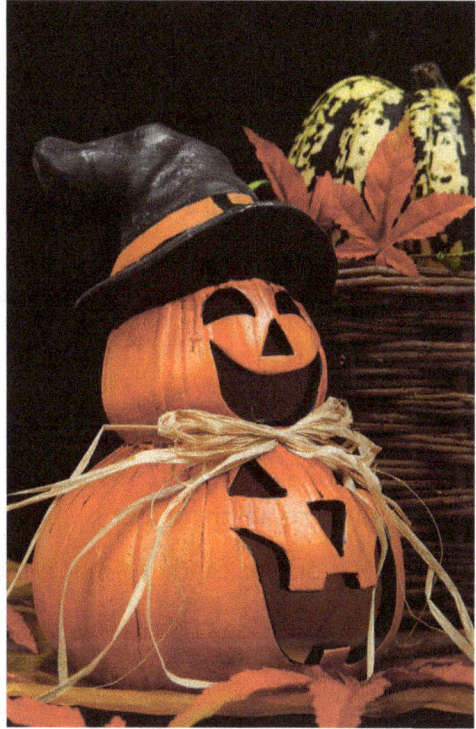

## Home Safe Home

- Clear a path to your door to avoid tripping a child

- Keep pathway and doorway well lit

- Restrain pets that may cause harm to a child

## Carving a Niche:

- Adults, not children, should carve the pumpkin. Children can scoop out the insides and draw a face on the pumpkin.

- Use a battery powered light inside of a pumpkin in place of a candle. Don't use an open flame for any decoration.

## Healthy Halloween:

- Give your youngsters a good meal before they collect all their sweet goodies

- Upon returning home, a responsible adult should inspect the treats and discard anything that is spoiled, unwrapped or suspicious

- Ration the candy so that it may be enjoyed for many days following Halloween

Have a happy and safe Halloween.

# Christmas Holiday Safety

With the holidays upon us, I wanted to take this opportunity to talk about holiday safety. I will discuss just a few of the many recommended safety precautions.

Poisoning:  Contrary to popular thought, the poinsettia plant is not poisonous, but if ingested could make a little one quite sick. Mistletoe and holly are considered poisonous. Be careful with these plants.

Choking:  Children have a natural tendency to put things in their mouths. The following are items to keep away from little children:  small toys or larger toys that can be broken down into smaller pieces, small batteries, small decorations and ornaments, coins, and food such as peanuts, popcorn, and small hard candy. Clean up carefully after opening presents as little ones can choke on scrap pieces of tape, wrapping paper, and ribbons. Look carefully around your living environment, and  be aware of children's exposure to anything that will fit in their mouths.

Burns:  Place candles in a safe location far from the reach of a young child, as well as away from flammable objects, such as curtains, decorations, and the good old Christmas tree. Keep matches and cigarette lighters out of a child's sight and reach. Do not leave burning candles unattended, and especially remember to extinguish them before going to bed. Have a fireguard in front of the fireplace. Do not burn wrapping paper in fireplaces, and be sure that the area around the fireplace is free of combustible material. Look around closely for potential fire hazards. Keep hot drinks and food out of a child's reach.

Injuries:  Check new and existing furniture, TVs, and equipment, to be sure they cannot be tipped over easily. Ensure that outdoor play equipment is assembled properly and has a soft surface underneath. I can't stress enough the importance of children wearing

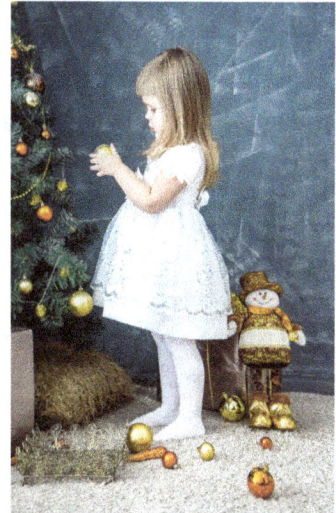

a helmet when riding bikes, scooters, etc. Too many children are seriously injured or killed from a head injury which could have easily been prevented by wearing a helmet.

Tree safety:  Make sure at time of purchase that an artificial tree is labeled "fire resistant". When purchasing a live tree be sure it is as fresh as possible. This can be done by shaking the tree to see if an over abundant number of needles fall off. Place the tree in a secure stand with water as soon as possible to keep it from further drying. Do not position it close to heat sources, such as fireplaces, heating  vents, and radiators. Use only flame resistant or non-flammable decorations to adorn the tree.

And now a word to adults. Christmas is a fun and social season, when a fair amount of alcohol and salty food can be consumed. A bit of over indulgence can cause "holiday heart" syndrome, which is due to an abnormal heart rhythm manifested by a fast and irregular heart beat. People with a history of atrial fibrillation are more susceptible to this condition, which although serious, is usually not life threatening. If it lasts more than a few hours, or if you feel short of breath, have chest pain, or feel  faint, go to the emergency room. And please, if you decide to enjoy alcoholic beverages, do not drive. Have a designated driver. Being in an accident or arrested for drunk driving is just not worth it.

Have a very happy and healthy holiday season.

## Autism

Autism is a developmental problem that appears early in childhood. It affects a child's social interaction, language, and behavior. This can make it difficult for an autistic child to communicate and interact with others.

Up to 6 out of every 1,000 children in the U.S. are diagnosed with autism and the numbers seem to be rising. This fact could be due to an actual increase in the incidence of autism, or perhaps is just a reflection of better detecting and reporting of the condition.

Diagnosis is difficult. Although the signs of autism may show up by 18 months of age, the diagnosis may not be reached until the age of 2 to 3 years. Early diagnosis is associated with a better chance of improvement.

Common symptoms of autism are:

- Social Skills: May not respond to his or her name, has poor eye contact, appears not to hear you, and retreats to his or her own world.

- Language: Starts talking later than other children, no eye contact when speaking, can't start a conversation or keep one going, and loses previously learned ability to say words or phrases.

- Behavior: Performs repetitive movements, develops strict routines and rituals, moves constantly, and is disturbed by the slightest change of routine.

There are many possible causes of autism including:

- Genetics:  Some genes are inherited and some can change after birth

- Environmental factors:  Environmental pollutants and virus infections may play a role in triggering autism

- Other causes:  Problems during labor and delivery at the time of birth, and possible adverse effects of the immune system may cause autis.

- Immunizations:  This is the greatest controversy, and a major reason why parents choose not to have their children routinely immunized. After much extensive study, to date, no link has been found between immunizations and autism.

Risk factors include:

- Childs sex:  Autism is 3 to 4 times more common in boys than girls
- Family history:  Families with one autistic child run a higher risk for having a second child with the disorder
- Paternal age:  The older the father, the greater chance of having an autistic child

Treatment of autism may include:

- Behavior and communication therapy
- Educational therapy
- Drug therapy (may help symptoms, but is not a cure)
- Creative therapy, such as music and art.

Coping with autism:

- Find a team of professionals who you can trust
- Learn as much as you can about the disorder
- Seek out other families of autistic children

We, as a community, need to be understanding and supportive of families with autistic children. Working with a child that requires extra attention can be exhausting for families. Autistic children can also bring talents beyond expectation. We can be grateful for such famous autistic geniuses as Beethoven, Mozart, and Einstein and the intricate world they shared with us.

# Down Syndrome

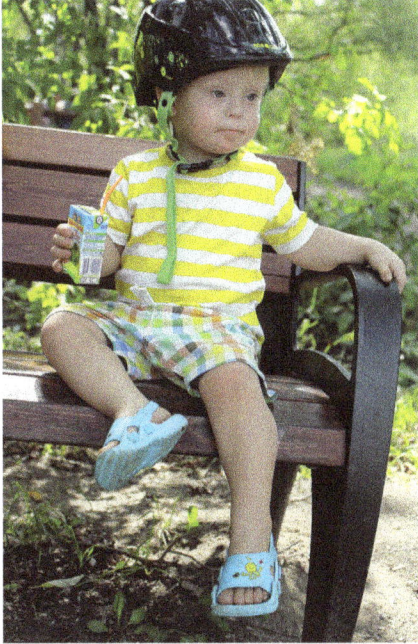

Down syndrome has particular meaning to me, because when I married my dear wife, Beth, I gained not only a wonderful wife, but also an equally incredible brother-in-law named Danny, who has Down syndrome. Coincidentally, Danny had been a patient of mine in urgent care for a number of years before I met Beth. I always enjoyed seeing him back then, as I already had a special affection for those with this genetic disorder.

Years ago while in medical school, I began a Sunday school class for the mentally handicapped most of whom had Down syndrome. I came away from that experience with a deep appreciation for these kids, little knowing that someday I would have one as a brother.

Danny has taught me some valuable lessons in life. Most importantly, he has shown to me what unconditional love is. I truly feel that he loves me, not for what I can do for him, but simply because I am his brother. I see in him a life free of the pressures and problems that affect so many of us. Granted, we don't live in a perfect world, but I see through Danny's life what it could be like if we were blessed to be free of the judgment of others and to be truly humble. This is not to say that he lacks feelings. I most often see him with a big grin on his face. And I've seen him cry and get angry. He can express himself like anyone else

He has a girlfriend, Jenni, who also has Down syndrome.  They met as toddlers 40 years ago, and their relationship endures. That's a much better track record than most marriages today.

Down syndrome is a genetic disorder with an abnormality of one of the chromosomes. It is named after John L. Down, a British doctor, who was the first to describe the syndrome back in the 1860's. It occurs in about 1 in 700 births.

Most people with Down syndrome share similar traits:

- Physical characteristics
- Delayed developmental milestones
- Some degree of mental retardation

Risks factors for having a Down syndrome baby are:

- Advancing maternal age
- Having had one child with Down syndrome
- Being a genetic carrier (rare)

Some people still believe that a child with Down syndrome should be in special education schools or even institutionalized. This couldn't be further from the truth. Most of those with Down syndrome live with their families or even independently. Some are able to be mainstreamed into regular schools through special education programs where they learn to read and write along with other curriculum. Some are able to hold down jobs.

It is my sincere hope that everyone can appreciate that a person with Down syndrome is as much of a human being as anyone else and deserves our love and respect. Parents, please talk to your kids about this and educate them about Down syndrome. The next time you see someone with Down syndrome give them a hearty smile, and don't be surprised if they shake your hand and a give you a big hug.

## Sugar in Our Diet

The average American consumes a whopping two to three pounds of sugar a week, or about 130 pounds a year. That's up from 25 pounds just 20 years ago. This rapid increase in consumption is because sugar is being increasingly added to many of our daily foods, such as soda, breakfast cereal, bread, mayonnaise, peanut butter, salad dressing, canned foods, and many other food products.

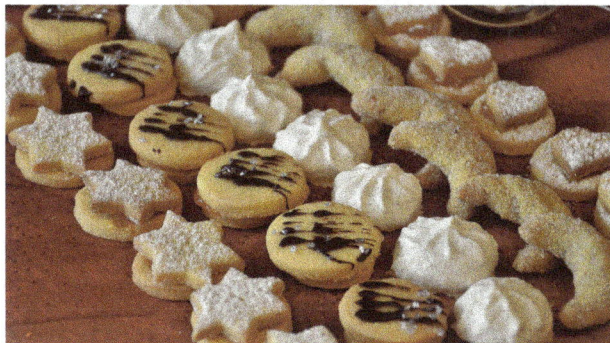

The main problem of eating too much sugar is that it adds extra calories to our diet, in most cases, much more than we need. Extra calories add up to weight gain and eventually to obesity, which is currently one of our greatest health epidemics. It is obesity from eating too much sugar, which can cause health problems such as diabetes, high blood pressure, heart attacks, and strokes.

Sugar is the main cause for dental cavities and tooth decay. It is also associated with an increase in triglycerides (a type of fat in the bloodstream), which can be another cause for heart disease.

There are many other possible but not necessarily proven health problems related to excessive dietary sugar, such as suppressing the immune system, hyperactivity in children, arthritis, asthma, and many more diseases.

Some think that natural sugar, such as found in fruits, dairy products, and other foods, is healthy. This is true only to the extent that these foods also contain healthy amounts of vitamins, fiber, and other nutrients.

Sugar is sugar no matter what it's called. There is brown sugar, high fructose corn syrup, dextrose, glucose, lactose, maltose, sucrose, molasses, honey, and others. They all contribute calories.

The American Heart Association says that women should get no more than 100 calories a day from added sugars. That's about 7 teaspoons or 25 grams, which is about equal to one typical candy bar. Men should get no more than 150 calories from sugar. That's about 10 teaspoons or 38 grams, the amount found in 12 ounces of soda. Most Americans get more than 22 teaspoons, or 355 calories, of added sugar a day, far exceeding healthy guidelines.

The best way to cut back on added sugar is to limit, if not eliminate, soft drinks from your diet. Many other drinks are high in sugar, including ready to drink teas, sweetened alcoholic or caffeine drinks, and juice drinks. To satisfy sweet cravings, try eating fresh fruit. For snacks, swap candy and sweets for air dried popcorn, dry roasted nuts, and baked tortilla chips.

Look at food labels which will list the ingredients, and often give the amount of sugar as measured in grams.

The bottom line is that most of us consume enough sugar naturally in a well balanced diet. The more we can cut back on candy, sodas, pastries, cakes, and cookies, the healthier we will be.

# Water Requirements

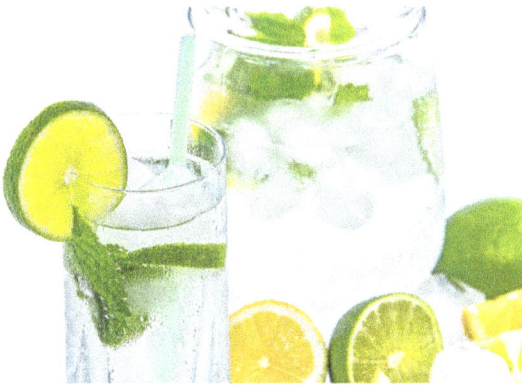

I'm often asked by patients how much water they need to drink each day. The Institute of Medicine has calculated that men need about 13 cups or 3 quarts of liquids and women need about 9 cups or 2 quarts of liquids daily. We also ingest approximately 2½ cups, or 20% of our daily intake of liquids from food, especially fruits and vegetables. In addition, beverages that we commonly drink such as coffee, juice, milk, and soda are composed mostly of water.

Water makes up 60% of our body weight. Every cell and system of our body depends on water. Lack of water causes dehydration, a condition that occurs when the body receives an inadequate amount of fluids, which in turn slows down and eventually shuts down vital bodily functions.

Our bodies constantly lose water from perspiring, breathing, urinating and having bowel movements.

Various factors determine just how much more water we may need to drink, such as:

- Environment – Hot weather, especially with high humidity, increases perspiration. Even in frigid weather, water is lost from our bodies when breathing during activities, such as skiing or hiking.

- Exercise –Also increases perspiration. The more prolonged and intense the exercising the greater the fluid loss.

- Illness – Intense or prolonged vomiting and/or diarrhea can lead to life threatening dehydration. This is an unfortunate cause of death in many developing countries.

- Pregnancy and breast feeding – Increases women's fluids needs

After hours of prolonged exercise with heavy sweating, we lose electrolytes, especially salt. This is when drinking a sports drink is recommended because it will not only replace the lost water, but also the depleted electrolytes. Electrolytes lost through sweat from mild to moderate exercise can be replaced from the food we eat.

Some liquids can act as a diuretic, which means they cause you to urinate more liquid than you've taken in. Caffeine is often implicated, but is really a weak diuretic. Alcoholic beverages on the other hand, especially at higher quantities, can be very potent diuretics causing dehydration, which is a major cause of a hangover.

A rough guide as to whether or not you are consuming enough water is to check your urine color. If it appears light yellow, like lemonade, you're probably well hydrated, and if it is very dark yellow, like apple juice, you need to drink more water.

To keep your body healthy:

- Drink a glass of water or other low or non-calorie beverage with each meal and between each meal
- Drink water before, during, and after exercise
- Or, do what makes sense and just follow the simple common advice to drink water when you're thirsty

# Radon

Radon is an odorless, colorless, radioactive gas found in the earth's crust throughout the world. It is formed from the breakdown of radioactive elements, such as uranium. Radon gas can move upward into the air and into underground and surface water. It dissipates in outside air where it causes no problems, but can be quite problematic if it seeps up into the house.

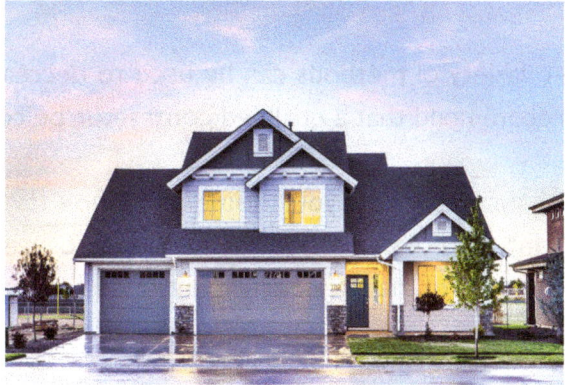

Any home can have an elevated radon level. New homes, old homes, well sealed or drafty, and with or without basements or crawl spaces. People who spend much of their time in basement rooms at home or at work have a greater risk of being exposed. Nearly one in fifteen homes has an elevated radon level. Radon levels cannot be predicted. They must be measured. The average radon level is 1.3 picocuries which is safe. A level above 4 picocuries is above the acceptable limit and needs to be dealt with.

Radon is the second leading cause of lung cancer in the U.S., causing an estimated 21,000 lung cancer deaths per year. Only smoking causes a greater percentage of lung cancer. Stop smoking and reduce your radon exposure to significantly lower your odds for lung cancer.

Radon gas decays into radioactive particles, which can get trapped in your lungs when breathing. These particles release small bursts of energy causing the damage to the lung tissue leading to cancer over a period of time. Not everyone exposed to such levels of radon will develop cancer, but many will without any idea it's happening.

As far as is known, radon exposure by itself, causes no obvious short term symptoms, unless it turns into symptoms of cancer, with shortness of breath, pain, or tightness in the chest, a worsening cough, and trouble breathing or swallowing.

You can check radon levels in your home. Do it yourself measuring kits can be bought, relatively inexpensively, at most hardware stores or online. The kits are placed in the home for several days then mailed to a lab for analysis.

A variety of methods can be used to decrease radon levels in the house if necessary. I recommend that a qualified contractor be contacted to get the job done correctly.

In summary, test your home for radon levels. If necessary, work with a professional contractor to decrease the radon exposure, quit smoking, and see your doctor if you have any of the previously mentioned signs of lung cancer.

## Advance Directives

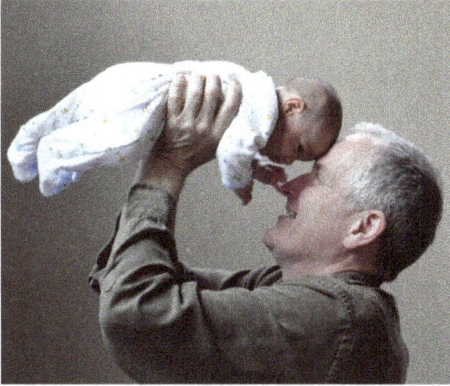

None of us ever would want to be incapacitated to the extent that we could not make decisions affecting our well-being. Unfortunately, for some of us that day may come. For most individuals, that time comes later in life, but for others it can happen much too early.

What sort of medical situations could cause such a scenario? You can be incapacitated by accident or illness, such as serious head injury, heart attack, stroke, Alzheimer's disease, meningitis, or by many other illnesses, diseases, and injuries.

To help in these situations, California has established a program called advance directives (sometimes referred to as "living wills"), which direct physicians as to your wishes for medical treatment if you were to be incapacitated and unable to make decisions on your own.

Under California law, there is a form called the Advance Health Care Directive. Some two-thirds of adults in the U.S. do not have this directive. With this form you may name an agent (power of attorney) who will make health care decisions on your behalf should you become incapacitated. This should be a trusted person also known as a proxy, and can be either a family member or friend. This person is one who has your best interests at heart, understands your wishes, and will act accordingly. Two alternates may also be named.

The directive must also be dated and executed in the presence of, and then signed by, two witnesses or by a notary. A witness cannot be your physician, any of his/her employees, or any employee of a health care facility. At least one of the witnesses cannot be related by blood, marriage, or adoption, and not be entitled to any part of your estate upon your death.

The most important function of the directive will permit health care providers to either prolong or not to prolong your life, and to keep you pain free according to your wishes. You may also state your desire for organ donation if you so choose.

Be sure that your chosen proxy and other important people in your life, such as your spouse, lawyer, adult children, and doctor, have copies of the form or know how to obtain it. Keep a copy in the home that is readily accessible by others.

It is important to make such decisions when you are of healthy mind and body. Don't put your loved ones in the difficult position of guessing what type of care you would want in an end of life event.

All adults need advance directives. Talk to your physician if you have any questions and also ask about the POLST (physician orders for life sustaining treatment) form. This a document created by you and your doctor that informs emergency care providers what kinds of treatments you want or don't want in a medical emergency. It is a medical order that must be followed by doctors, hospital personnel, and paramedics. It is intended to complement and not replace the health care directive.

If you live in a state other than California, consult your physician regarding your state's guidelines on health care directives.

# Alzheimer's

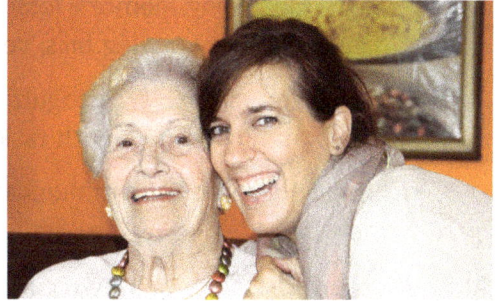

Alzheimer's disease is the most common form of dementia, which is a term for loss of memory and other mental abilities severe enough to interfere with daily life. It is caused by physical changes within the brain. It was first described in the early 1900's by Dr. Alois Alzheimer, and is a progressive, irreversible brain disorder causing severe memory loss, difficulty thinking, and eventually robbing a person of being able to perform even the simplest of tasks.

Over five million people in the U.S are living with Alzheimer's disease, and it is the seventh leading cause of death. It afflicts one in eight people age 65 and older, and one in two people over age 85. Very few families are untouched by this disease.

Our brains, as well as all organs in our bodies change as we age. Slower thinking and some memory loss occur to some extent in all of us the longer we live. Serious memory loss, confusion, and inability to perform simple tasks are not normal, but reflect a more severe deterioration of our brain cells, of which there are over 100 billion in the average adult brain.

The cause of Alzheimer's disease is unknown, but it is thought to be associated with genetic, lifestyle, and environmental factors.

Abnormal structures called plaques and tangles have been identified in and around brain cells in those patients who have Alzheimer' disease. They are thought to block communication between cells and lead to their destruction. Unlike other cells in our body, brain cells regenerate very slowly, if at all, thus the continued progression of Alzheimer's disease.

Various stages of Alzheimer's disease have been identified and are described as:

- Early: Increasing memory problems only
- Mild: Increasing memory loss with problems such as getting lost, trouble handling money, paying bills, repeating questions, and poor judgment
- Moderate: Difficulty recognizing family and friends, unable to learn new things, having trouble with tasks, such as getting dressed
- Severe: Unable to communicate and completely dependent on others for their care

Although there is as yet no known cure for Alzheimer's disease, several drugs have been approved for the treatment of the symptoms. These drugs help to maintain memory, thinking, and some behavioral skills, but they don't change the disease process and may only help for a few months to a few years.

Be proactive to help prevent Alzheimer's disease by:

- Keeping cholesterol level normal or below
- Boosting your vitamin D level by sun exposure, appropriate foods, or vitamin supplements
- Exercising your brain playing cards or doing crossword puzzles
- Maintaining social contact with friends and family
- Keeping physically active

Those who are close to someone with Alzheimer's disease understand the tremendous toll it takes emotionally, physically, and financially. Caregivers can be helped by developing a support network of family and friends. Organized support groups such as The Alzheimer's Association (www.alz.org) are also available, and can offer much needed help and advice for those who are caring for someone with Alzheimer's disease.

# Falls in the Elderly

Falls are the leading cause of injury related emergency room visits in persons over 65 years of age. The risk of falling increases with age and is greater for women than men. Falls are the leading cause of death from injury among the elderly. Almost 10,000 deaths in older Americans are caused by falls every year. The most significant consequence of falling is the loss of independence. After a serious fall, an elderly person often suffers a decline in normal activities of daily living, and is often permanently placed in an assisted living facility or in a nursing home.

Hip fractures are a frequent consequence of falls and occur to more than 250,000 elderly people, at a health care cost of approximately 10 billion dollars each year. Twenty five percent of those who sustain a hip fracture require life-long nursing home care. Other injuries from a fall include head injuries, lacerations, severe bruising, and fractures of arms or legs.

Risk factors of falls and preventative measures are as follows:

Impaired vision:

- Have regular vision checkups
- Add contrasting colored strips on the edges of first and last steps to identify change of level

Lack of physical activity:

- Exercise regularly to maintain muscle tone and strength

Osteoporosis:

- Work with your doctor to diagnosis and treat osteoporosis (thinning of the bones)

Medications:

- Prescription pain medicine, sedatives, and anti depressant drugs are the biggest medication culprits in causing falls

- Beware of alcohol interacting with drugs

- Know the common side effects of your medications

Home hazards:

- Avoid throw rugs

- Reduce clutter

- Maintain adequate lighting

- Install grab bars around tub and toilet

- Keep commonly used items in easy reach

- Avoid using floor polish or wax in order to prevent slipping

- Remove caster wheels from furniture

- Use night lights

- Avoid step-stools and ladders

I would love to start a campaign to have our society remove all concrete parking bumpers in parking lots. They are accidents waiting to happen. The elderly tend to fall face first onto the pavement as I have witnessed all too many times in my practice. Please be extremely careful when walking to and from your car to avoid tripping over these bumper hazards.

As we age, we all need to move around more carefully and slow things down a bit to prevent falls, and to help us enjoy a longer, healthier, and independent life.

# Palliative/Hospice Care

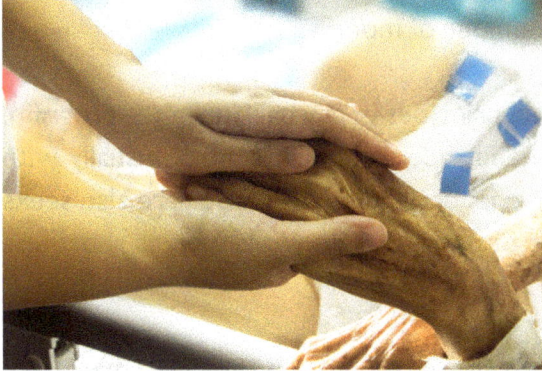

There seems to be some confusion when it comes to understanding the difference between palliative care and hospice. They are both distinctive medical disciplines and often work together.

Hospice care comes into play when a patient has a terminal illness and all treatment options have been exhausted. It is really for those who have been determined to be in their last six months of life. The goal of hospice care is not to cure the underlying disease, but to support the quality of life. Hospice care is usually provided by a team of health care professionals who maximize comfort for terminally ill patients, while also addressing physical, social, and spiritual needs.

Hospice care is most commonly provided at a patient's home, with a family member typically serving as the primary caregiver. It is often available wherever the patient is, whether at hospitals, nursing homes, or assisted living facilities. The hospice care team is usually available 24 hours a day, 7 days a week.

Palliative care is medical care based on the goal to relieve pain and suffering, reduce symptoms, ease stress, and mainly to improve a patient's quality of life during a serious illness and is not limited to end of life issues. People who are actively being treated for a disease can receive palliative care at any stage of their illness, whereas hospice is thought of as end of life care.

This is an important distinction because many people think of palliative care as end of life care and therefore is often not requested when it's most needed and helpful. Recent studies are showing the benefits of beginning palliative care soon after the diagnosis of a serious illness, or when an ongoing illness worsens.

The palliative care team works closely with the patient's primary treating physician in caring for the patient. While the patient's treating physicians may be trying to prolong life, palliative care's goal is to maximize quality of life. It has been shown that palliative care can actually extend a patient's life for a number of months.

Identifying and managing pain is one of the main priorities of any palliative care program. Cancer is the most common disease which needs adequate pain control, usually with opiate drugs like oxycodone and morphine, and its derivatives. Palliative care also seeks to improve many other troublesome sources of physical discomfort such as shortness of breath, constipation, and insomnia.

With the help of a social worker, palliative care also deals with psychological and social services both for the patients and their caregivers, as well as helping with practical problems, such as coordinating doctors visits and arranging transportation.

Talk with your physician for further information.

Have you ever had any of these experiences?

- You walk into a room and forget what you wanted to do

- You want to drive somewhere but you can't remember where you left the car keys

- You're shopping and you see one of your close neighbors but you can't remember their name

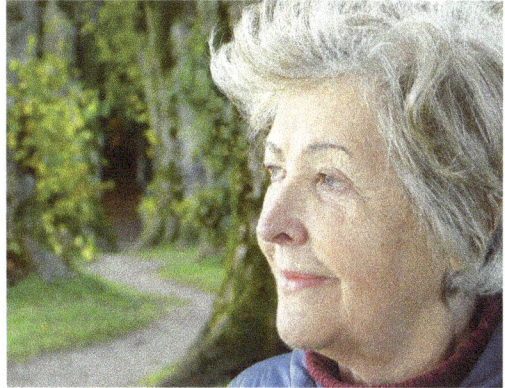

These are but a few examples of what are commonly referred to as senior moments. Many people who have these forgetful moments fear that they may be in the early stages of Alzheimer's disease, but the fact is that almost everyone, especially starting around the age of 50, has these experiences.

Factors that can worsen memory loss are:

- Lack of sleep

- Uncontrolled high blood pressure

- Excessive use of alcohol

- Medications

- Loneliness, anxiety, and depression

Just as aging affects our bodies, it also causes changes in our brains. Memory lapses are some of the more obvious changes that we will all experience. Although we can't keep our brains from physically aging, we can be proactive to slow down those changes.

The following are my recommendations to keeping our brains as healthy as possible as we age:

- Concentrate, pay attention, and use mental images to help remember things
- Maintain a positive attitude and continue to find purpose in life
- Remain physically active with some form of regular exercise
- Stimulate the brain by doing puzzles, word games, reading, and conversing
- Maintain adequate sleep. A regular brief nap is very beneficial.
- Eat a healthy balanced diet
- Avoid alcohol or at least limit its use
- Get organized. Use calendars, notes, and lists to jog the memory.
- Do not isolate yourself. Remain socially active with family and friends.
- Relax through yoga, meditation, and prayer

The bottom line is that we all experience occasional memory loss. This is part of the normal aging process. Senior moments usually cause only minor annoyances, occasional slips, and inconvenience, and are no cause for worry or concern. If your moments become persistent, worsen, or interfere with daily activities, you should see your doctor so that your symptoms can be evaluated.

When it comes to caring for your brain my advice is "use it or lose it."

## Diabetes Part 1

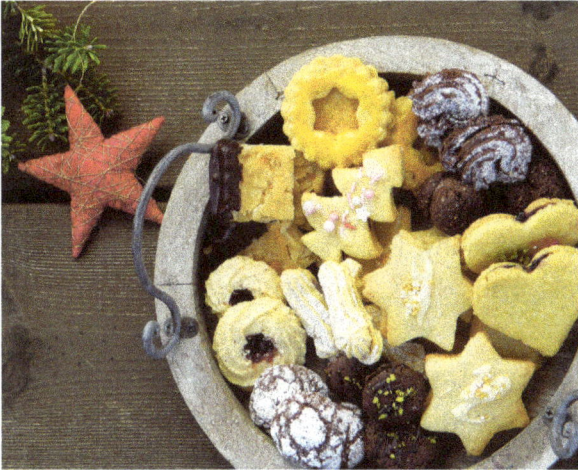

Most of us know someone with diabetes but we may not understand just what this disease is. Diabetes occurs when the body doesn't make enough insulin or when the insulin becomes ineffective. Insulin is a hormone made by the pancreas, which helps move glucose (blood sugar) from the blood into the cells of our bodies, where the glucose acts as a source of life sustaining energy for our muscles and tissues. When insulin is insufficient or ineffective, the sugar level in our blood increases, causing diabetes.

There are several types of diabetes. In type 1 diabetes, one's pancreas does not produce enough insulin. This is usually caused by a genetic or environmental problem, when one's own immune system attacks and destroys the cells that create insulin in the pancreas. This type of diabetes often starts in childhood and has the most serious health complications.

Type 2 diabetes occurs when one's cells become resistant to the effects of insulin causing sugar to build up in the bloodstream. Being overweight is a major contributing factor. Genetics and environmental factors may also play a role in this type of diabetes. Type 2 diabetes is the most common type, occurring at any age.

Prediabetes often precedes type 2 diabetes. This condition occurs when the blood sugar is higher than normal, but not high enough to cause any obvious health problems. It is estimated that some 80 million people in the U.S. have this condition, which if not recognized and treated, could go on to type 2 diabetes.

Symptoms of diabetes depend on how high one's blood sugar is and includes:

- Frequent urination
- Increased thirst
- Extreme hunger
- Unexplained weight loss

Risk factors for diabetes depend on the type of diabetes. For type I these factors include: genetics, environmental, dietary, race and geography. Risk factors for type 2 include: obesity, inactivity, family history, age, and pregnancy.

Complications of diabetes take time to develop. The longer one has diabetes and the higher the blood sugar the worse the complication. Eventually these complications can cause significant disability and possible early death. Diabetic complications include:

- Cardiovascular disease, especially heart attacks and strokes
- Nerve (neuropathy) and blood vessel damage involving the legs and feet sometimes leading to amputation
- Eye damage
- Kidney damage, often leading to dialysis or even to kidney transplantation
- Increased risk of Alzheimer's disease, as well as certain cancers

# Diabetes Part 2

I would like to discuss the diagnostic tests, treatments, prevention, and the impact of diabetes on our society.

Blood tests are used to diagnose diabetes. The fasting blood sugar test is the one most commonly used. It tests the amount of sugar in the bloodstream after a period of fasting. A more reliable blood test is called the AIC test and measures the average blood sugar over the past several months.

Specific treatment for type 1 diabetes involves the use of insulin, frequent monitoring of one's blood sugar level, and counting carbohydrates. Treatment of type 2 diabetes involves oral diabetes medications, possible use of insulin, blood sugar monitoring, maintaining a proper diet, and routine exercise.

Type 1 diabetes can't be prevented, and can only be treated with insulin. However, type 2 diabetes can be prevented by the same lifestyle choices that also treat this condition, including:

- Eating healthy foods
- Getting plenty of physical activity
- Losing extra pounds if overweight

Some 26 million Americans have diabetes and the numbers are growing yearly. Approximately 2 million of these diabetics have type 1 diabetes, and the remaining 24 million have the more preventable type 2 diabetes. 26% of all hospital costs are related to the treatment of diabetes and its complications, costing some $175-$200 billion per year.

In summary, we know that type 1 diabetes usually begins in childhood, is most often caused by genetic or other unknown factors, is not caused by a poor diet, and is not caused by "eating too much sugar." Type 1 (childhood) diabetes is caused by the body not having enough insulin, which causes increased blood sugar. It is treated with insulin injections. Also such an afflicted child will not "grow out of it." Type 1 diabetes is a lifetime health issue.

Type 2 diabetes affects mostly adults and is treated and often cured by diet, exercise, and preventing obesity.

25 million Americans have prediabetes (a precursor to diabetes). I would advise patients to talk with their physicians at their next routine visit about being screened for this common disease.

# Osteoporosis

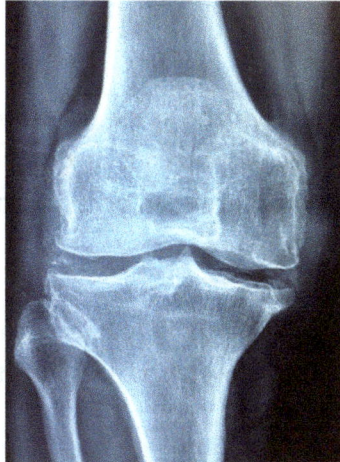

Osteoporosis literally means "bones with holes." It occurs when bone loses calcium faster than it can be replaced. New bone creation doesn't keep pace with the removal of old bone. The bone is weaker, less dense, and easier to break than is healthy bone.

Common unchangeable risk factors for osteoporosis are:

- Your sex: Women, especially post menopausal, are much more likely to develop osteoporosis then men, but men aren't off the hook. There are at least 2 million men with osteoporosis, and this will increase as men begin to live longer.

- Age: The older the age, the greater the chance of developing osteoporosis

- Family history. You're at a greater risk if any close relatives have had osteoporosis

- Race: Caucasian and Asian women are at a greater risk

The reduction of sex hormones, estrogen for women and testosterone for men, also contributes to osteoporosis. Dietary factors associated with osteoporosis include low calcium intake, eating disorders, and stomach bypass surgery. Certain medications, especially corticosteroids such as prednisone and cortisone, can contribute to osteoporosis.

Lifestyle choices also can put you at a greater risk for osteoporosis:

- Sedentary lifestyle. Lack of exercise.
- Excessive alcohol consumption, especially more than 2 drinks a day
- Tobacco use

Bone fractures, especially of the hip and spine, are the most common complications of osteoporosis. A fall can easily break a hip causing disability and even complications in the elderly, leading to death. Spinal fractures can occur with or without an injury. Sometimes a sneeze or cough can cause a fracture.

The best way to diagnose osteoporosis is to measure bone density. This can be done by a machine that uses low levels of x-ray to measure the strength of your bones. Your doctor can order this for you.

Osteoporosis can be treated with drugs called biophosphonates. Your doctor would have a choice of one of several of these drugs to treat you. Use of the sex hormones estrogen for women and testosterone for men can also be useful in treating osteoporosis. Some controversy exists over the use of these hormones. Your doctor will explain the risks and benefits.

Here are suggestions that may help reduce your risk of developing osteoporosis:

- Avoid excessive alcohol
- Don't smoke
- Try to avoid falls
- Exercise regularly
- Consume adequate amounts of calcium. It is recommended that the total daily calcium intake from diet or supplements not exceed 2,000 mg. daily for people over age 50.
- Consume adequate amounts of vitamin D. This is necessary for your body to absorb calcium. Talk to your doctor about what dose would be best for you.

# Thyroid Disease

The thyroid gland which is located in the front of your neck below the Adam's apple, makes thyroid hormones. These hormones help regulate the heart rate, body temperature, the conversion of food into energy, and the control our metabolism.

Malfunctioning of the thyroid gland can cause several well known conditions. Sometimes the gland doesn't manufacture enough thyroid hormone, a condition called hypothyroidism, which in turn causes parts of the body to not function normally. Symptoms of this include feeling tired, always feeling cold, having a slow heart rate, dry skin, constipation, weight gain, muscle weakness, and achiness. Without treatment, these symptoms slowly become more severe. Constant stimulation of the thyroid gland to release more hormones may lead to an enlarged thyroid known as a goiter.

Causes of hypothyroidism include autoimmune disease where your own immune system produces antibodies that attack and destroy thyroid tissue, prior treatment for hyperthyroidism, thyroid surgery, certain medications, and radiation.

Risk factors of hypothyroidism include being a female over 65 years of age, a family history of thyroid disease, having an auto immune disease, prior treatment with radioactive iodine, and having been pregnant or delivered a baby in the past 6 months.

Standard treatment for hypothyroidism involves daily use of the synthetic thyroid hormone levothyroxine (Levothroid, Synthroid, others). This oral medication restores adequate hormone levels, reversing the signs and symptoms of hypothyroidism.

Hyperthyroidism is when the thyroid gland produces too much of the thyroid hormone called thyroxin. Common symptoms of this condition include unexplained sudden weight loss, a rapid irregular heart rate, nervousness, increased appetite, heat sensitivity, fatigue, muscle weakness, skin thinning, and fine brittle hair.

Causes of hyperthyroidism include Grave's disease, an autoimmune disorder in which our own immune system stimulates the thyroid gland to produce too much thyroid hormone. Also a condition known as thyroiditis causes an increase in hormone production due to the thyroid gland becoming inflamed for unknown reasons.

Treatment for hyperthyroidism includes radioactive iodine, which when taken by mouth helps the gland to shrink and symptoms to subside. Anti-thyroid medications can also be taken by mouth to prevent the gland from over production of thyroid hormone. Beta blocker medication is used to control the symptoms of rapid heart rate and high blood pressure.

See your doctor regarding any of the above mentioned symptoms for proper evaluation and treatment and expect a likely referral to an endocrinologist (hormone specialist).

## Conjunctivitis

Pinkeye (medically known as conjunctivitis) is an inflammation or infection of the conjunctiva, which is the transparent thin tissue covering the surface of the eyeball and inner eyelids. This condition causes the affected eye or eyes to appear pink or even red because the tiny blood vessels on the surface of the eye become swollen thus causing the pink color.

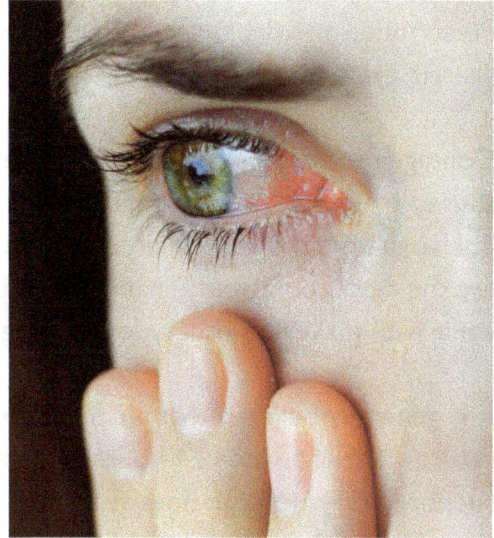

There are several causes of pinkeye. The most common form is caused by a virus infection which is often associated with a head cold. Virus pinkeye is highly contagious and passed on to others by direct contact with the patient and his or her secretions, or with contaminated objects or surfaces. Patients usually report awakening in the morning with a crusty mucous in their eyes and perhaps a small amount of mucous during the daytime. One may have the sensation of grittiness, burning, or just irritation. Usually both eyes are involved. Virus pinkeye will cure itself, no treatment is necessary. It has to run its course and is usually gone within one week but may take up to two weeks. Over the counter eye drops such as Naphcon-A may provide some relief of the symptoms.

Another form of infectious pinkeye is caused by a bacterial infection. This is usually not associated with the common cold and is more common in children than in adults. It is also very contagious and is spread as mentioned above in virus pinkeye. Patients with this infection often have just one eye involved, and it is usually "stuck shut" upon awakening. The affected eye or eyes usually produce a pus-like discharge throughout the entire day, which helps to differentiate it from virus pinkeye, which only has mucous upon awakening. Bacterial pinkeye is treatable with prescription antibiotic eye drops, which will usually clear up the infection within a few days.

Pinkeye can also be caused by allergies. This is usually due to airborne particles, such as pollen or cat dander. A patient with this form of pinkeye usually has both eyes affected, has an itchy feeling, and is likely to have some crusting of the eyes upon awakening. Prescription eye drops from your doctor are available for more severe and persistent allergic eye symptoms.

Contagiousness seems to be the greatest concern with pinkeye. The infectious varieties caused by either virus or bacteria are highly contagious from contact with the mucus discharge from the eye. Children who are too young to understand the concepts of hygiene are the most contagious. That is why it is so prevalent in preschool and kindergarten. An adult with pinkeye is usually less contagious because of practicing good hygiene.

It is generally believed that a child who has been placed on antibiotic eye medicine can return to school after 24 hours of treatment. Although there is no scientific proof to support this concept, it does seem to work. My personal bias is that a person with infectious pinkeye is contagious as long as there is discharge from the eyes.

Practicing good hygiene is the best way of limiting the spread of pinkeye. Once you have symptoms of an infection I suggest the following:

- Don't touch your eyes with your hands
- Wash your hands with soap and water thoroughly and frequently
- Don't share towels or face cloths with anyone
- Change to new eye cosmetics, especially mascara
- Follow your eye doctor's recommendation if you wear contact lenses

If you have any of the following symptoms, see your doctor immediately:

- Decreased vision
- Sensitivity to bright light
- Sensation of something painful in the eye

# Dizziness

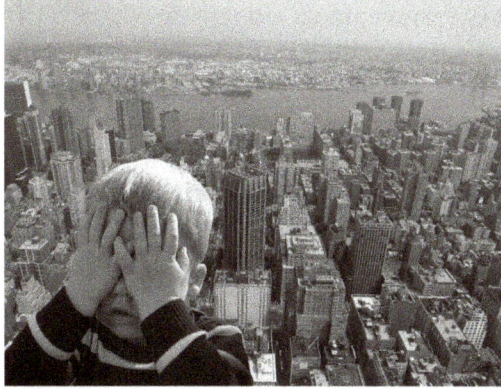

Dizziness is a term to describe a sensation of lightheadedness, loss of balance, feeling unsteady, or faint. Dizziness, which causes a feeling that you or the room is moving or spinning, is called vertigo. Although these symptoms may be incapacitating or disabling, dizziness is rarely a sign of a serious or life threatening condition.

Symptoms may also include nausea, vomiting, weakness, and fatigue. More serious symptoms prompting immediate emergency attention are: severe headache, high fever (above 101 degrees), stiff neck, visual or hearing loss, weakness of an arm or leg, and dizziness due to a head injury.

There are several classifications of dizziness:

- Lightheadedness – This is usually caused by a lack of sufficient blood getting to the brain. This can be due to very low blood pressure, an arrhythmia (irregular heart beat), dehydration, or a stroke.

- Loss of balance – Can be caused by an inner ear disturbance, failing vision, nerve damage in the legs, and by side effects of certain medications.

- Vertigo – There are several types:

    1. Benign paroxysmal positional vertigo (BPPV): This occurs when a tiny mineral particle gets stuck in a sensitive section of the semicircular canal, a fluid filled area of the inner ear that regulates our balance as we change

positions. This condition is brought about by movement or changing position of the head such as turning over in bed, or sitting up. Many patients with this condition can have almost instantaneous relief from a simple exercise of head movements done in a doctor's office. This treatment called the Epley manuever can be found on YouTube, and can be tried at home. This maneuver dislodges the offending particle thus eliminating the vertigo symptoms.

2.  Inflammation in the inner ear (labyrinthitis):  This can develop from a cold or an allergy and can cause sudden intense vertigo and can last several days. Unlike BPPV, this condition can happen any time and is not associated with movement of the head. An over the counter medication called Bonine can often give relief to symptoms from this disorder.

3.  Meniere's disease:  This is caused by a fluid accumulation in the inner ear. It is characterized by sudden episodes of intense vertigo with nausea and vomiting. Other symptoms may include hearing loss, and ringing or fullness in the ear. This is a more chronic condition and may need to be treated by an Ear Nose and Throat specialist.

Many patients I see with dizziness or vertigo symptoms fear they may be having a stroke or some other serious problem. Most of them have one of the above mentioned conditions, and can be treated either with the head positioning maneuvers or with medication. Thankfully, most of these conditions resolve on their own and when they don't, medical attention is needed.

# Ear Wax

I'm writing about a subject that may not be too appealing or romantic, but it's something that pretty much affects all of us. A frequent cause of hearing loss is blockage due to ear wax, also called *cerumen*.

Ear wax is actually not a wax, but a mixture of skin cells and oil secreted by glands in the ear canal. Its purpose is to lubricate and protect the sensitive lining of the canal. It has some antimicrobial properties, which means it can help to fight off infections.

Most of the time cerumen has a tendency, due to chewing and jaw movements, to move to the opening of the ear where it dries up and flakes out of the ear and disappears, causing no problems.

When an ear canal is blocked up with cerumen, it is called an impaction. This can occur when one produces an overabundance of ear wax, or can be caused by the use of a Q Tip which more often than not forces the cerumen deeper into the ear canal rather than cleaning it out. The use of a Q Tip can also scratch your ear canal and cause an infection. This is why it's often said not to stick anything in your ear "smaller than your elbow."

With a cerumen impaction, you will most likely feel a pressure sensation in your ear canal and experience some degree of hearing loss. These are the symptoms that will usually cause a patient to see their doctor.

Once your doctor looks in your ear and verifies the wax blockage, he or she has several options to remove it. The most common method used is to flush out the ear with pressurized water. Another method your doctor may use is to take a small wire instrument and, under direct vision, remove the wax manually.

There are ear wax removal kits found at pharmacies that contain wax softening drops and a bulb syringe to flush out the ear. Although not always successful, they're probably worth a try.

I advise my patients after the wax has been removed, to do some home therapy to prevent further wax buildup. Once a week, perhaps when bathing, they should flush out their ears with warm water, using a common rubber bulb syringe found at any pharmacy. This method should clean out any wax before it accumulates.

See your doctor for any persistent problems with hearing loss, pain, discharge from the ear, or any other worrisome symptoms.

# Earache

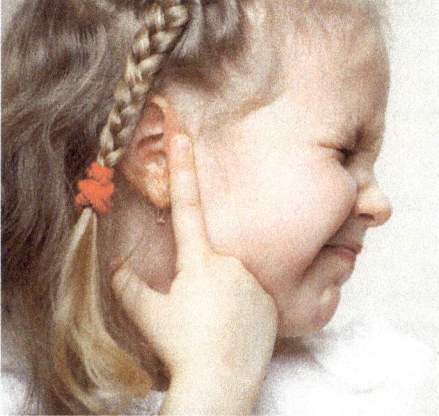

There are various reasons why one's ear can hurt. The most common reason is a condition called *otitis media*, an infection of the middle ear, which mostly affects children and occasionally adults. The baby or child who awakens crying in the middle of the night most likely has otitis media. It is one of the most common reasons that children are taken to their doctor.

The ear was designed to receive sound waves and transmit them to the brain. To understand ear infections, we must know a little about the anatomy of the normal ear. The outer ear is what is visible externally and also includes the ear canal (which is that portion of the ear into which we are not to put Q Tips!). The middle ear is the space behind the eardrum. The Eustachian tube connects the middle ear to the back of the nose and throat area. It functions to allow the pressure in the middle ear to change as the pressure around us changes. Sound waves set the eardrums vibrating sending impulses to the brain. The inner ear is like a tiny gyroscope, which deals with helping to maintain proper balance with our surroundings.

Middle ear infections usually occur from a blockage of the Eustachian tube from having a head cold or allergy. The tube blockage allows fluid to build up in the middle ear, which is a perfect setting for either bacteria or viruses to grow and cause the infection. This then increases the pressure behind the sensitive eardrum, which is what actually causes the pain.

This condition is more common in children than adults because the young Eustachian tube is shorter and smaller and therefore more easily blocked up. Middle ear infections can cause temporary hearing loss in children. Recurrent infections can cause more prolonged hearing loss and may cause some development of speech and language skills.

These recurrent infections can often be remedied by having an ear-nose-throat doctor put tiny tubes, called *tympanostomy tubes,* in the eardrum to allow the excessive fluid to be drained out of the middle ear. The tubes which are placed during a surgical procedure usually fall out on their own after many months.

The most common symptom of an ear infection is pain. This may be verbalized by an older child, or for a baby, this may be signaled by fussiness, irritability, or poor appetite. Fever is often but not always present. Sometimes the pressure becomes so great in the middle ear that the ear drum may burst (only a tiny hole), and there may be blood or pus draining from the ear. This is not dangerous to the child and will actually stop the pain by relieving the pressure built up in the middle ear. However, it is all the more reason to see your doctor for evaluation and treatment.

Treatment of otitis media often includes any of the following:

- Antibiotics have traditionally been routinely prescribed over the years. We have come to realize that these infections will often go away by themselves because they are usually caused by a virus. Even if caused by bacteria, it seems that the child's immune system may overcome the infection.  Antibiotics are usually prescribed initially in the very young and especially those who are in a day care setting.

- Pain relievers such as Tylenol or ibuprofen may be given to reduce both pain and fever. Giving the appropriate dose, and giving it regularly every 6 hours, seems to work best.

- A warm heating pad or compress held to the painful can be helpful.

- If the eardrum has burst, antibiotic ear drops are often prescribed.

Usually your doctor will want to see the child after treatment to make sure the infection has gone.

# Eye Diseases

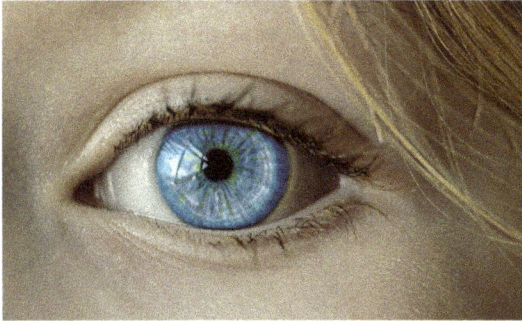

It is said that by age 75, a majority of us will be developing problems with our eyes that could lead to serious vision loss. At that age, more than one half of people will have cataracts, and around 20 percent will have either macular degeneration or glaucoma.

These diseases are all related to the aging process which of course we cannot change, but as I will explain, there are some things we can do to reduce the risk.

**Cataracts** – A condition caused by the clouding of the normally crystal clear lens of the eye. This results in hazy vision, increased visual glare, seeing halos around lights, and poor night vision. A cataract can develop in one or both eyes. Some risk factors that can cause cataracts are: increasing age, excessive exposure to sunlight, diabetes, drinking excessive alcohol, and smoking.

As the cataracts worsen, surgery will often become necessary. This involves removing the cloudy lens and replacing it with a plastic lens implant. This is routine surgery with minimal risk and great benefit.

**Macular degeneration** – This occurs with failure of the macula, which is in the center of our retina, and is responsible for clear vision. There are two types of degeneration. Dry macular degeneration is the most common and is caused by a thinning and breakdown of the macular tissue. Wet macular degeneration can progress from the dry variety and is due to leaky blood vessel around the macula and is often more serious. Both types can cause serious central blurring and even a central blind spot.

Treatment for dry macular degeneration involves taking antioxidant vitamins, and for the wet variety, there are new drugs that prevent the leaky blood vessels.

**Glaucoma** – This is caused by an increased pressure that builds up inside the eyeball. It results in damage to the optic nerve which then interferes with the transmission of images to the brain, resulting in severe loss of vision. Treatment begins with eye drops, which will usually need to be used for the rest of one's life. Several different surgical procedures are available for some types of glaucoma.

There are things you can do to help save your vision including:

- Wear sunglasses when outdoors during daylight

- Quit smoking

- Moderate alcohol consumption

- Control chronic diseases such as diabetes and hypertension

- Exercise regularly and eat a healthy diet with lots of fresh fruits and vegetables (I now realize that my mother was right when she told me during my childhood to eat lots of carrots to help my vision)

See your doctor immediately if you have any obvious visual change. People between the ages of 18 and 50 should have routine eye exams every 2 years and every year after the age of 50. Children need routine eye exams as well. Ask your child's doctor about the frequency.

# Hearing Loss

Are you having difficulty understanding words in a conversation, or turning up the volume on your TV, or asking people to repeat themselves when speaking to you, or even avoiding conversations and social gatherings? If so, you are likely suffering from hearing loss. Up to one third of those between the ages of 65 to 75, and one half of those over 75, have some degree of hearing loss.

Hearing loss can occur for a number of reasons:

- Prolonged exposure to loud noise. which damages the very sensitive inner ear nerves
- Earwax, which can build up in the ear canal and form a physical barrier blocking sound waves from the inner ear
- Ruptured eardrum from exposure to an explosive noise, from infection, or from damage, such as sticking something in your ear, most commonly a Q Tip

There are various risk factors leading to hearing loss including:

- Occupational or recreational noise
- Advancing age
- Heredity
- Side effects of some medications
- Result of infection such as meningitis or measles

Treatment and prevention for hearing loss include:

- Wear earplugs at concerts or when exposed to loud noise at home or work.
- Removing earwax when indicated.
- Hearing aids.
- Cochlear implants for more severe hearing loss

If you are suffering from hearing loss, I strongly urge you to consider a hearing aid. Technological advances have made hearing aids an excellent option to restore hearing. Many people are reluctant to use hearing aids. This may be due to a perceived negative stigma attached to hearing loss or to expense, since hearing aids can be expensive and not covered by Medicare or by most private insurances. Contrary to these fears, the use of hearing aids can significantly enhance social situations and provide a more enjoyable lifestyle, and may even delay early dementia.

If you are having problems with your hearing, make an appointment with a qualified audiologist and have a routine hearing test. From there you may be referred to an ear, nose, and throat doctor for treatment of a specific problem, or the audiologist may be able to provide you with an appropriate hearing aid. Don't put off what may be a life enhancing experience for you.

# Strep Throat

Sore throats are most commonly caused by an infection, usually by viruses, or occasionally by bacteria, such as the strep germ. The sore throat from a virus is by far the most common variety and is usually accompanied by cold-like symptoms, such as cough and runny nose. This type of sore throat is really just one of the many irritating symptoms of the cold virus, and will run its course without the need of antibiotics. It often lasts 3 to 10 days. It is rarely associated with a fever.

Strep throat is caused by the streptococcus bacteria and can often feel like just any other type of sore throat. It is most common in childhood and tapers off as one gets older. Some lucky people never get it, and some get it often. What's important and different about strep throat is that if it is left untreated with antibiotics, it can lead to rheumatic fever (a potentially serious disease affecting children from 5-15 years of age, but is very rare in the U.S). Strep throat can also cause a fine red rash on the body called scarlet fever, which has a very scary sound to it, but in reality it is just a non-serious rash that sometimes occurs with strep throat.

Symptoms of strep throat are sore throat, fever, tender swollen glands in the neck, and nausea or stomachache. A white coating on the throat is often a sign of strep but is not fool-proof because it can also be caused by viruses. There is usually not an associated runny nose or cough with strep throat.

Tonsillitis is an infection of the tonsils, which are the two glands found in your throat on either side of the back of the tongue. Healthy tonsils are usually not visible because they are so small. Tonsillitis is most common in childhood and can be caused by either the strep germ or by a virus. Tonsillectomy (surgical removal of the tonsils,) which was done routinely when I was a kid, is now only done in patients with repeated episodes of strep tonsillitis.

When you have a sore throat that concerns you, see your health provider who will listen to your symptoms, perform an examination, and will often order laboratory testing from a swab of your throat. The tests are usually a rapid test that takes about 10 minutes and is done in the office, and/or a culture that will be sent out to a lab taking about 24 to 48 hour for the results.

The treatment of choice for strep throat is penicillin, or its close relative, amoxicillin. Strep is one of the few infections where penicillin is still the best cure. People will usually feel better within 1-2 days after beginning treatment. A child being treated for strep can usually return to school within 1-2 days if there is no fever and if feeling well enough. A prescription for 10 days is usually given, and it is important to take it to the last pill, even when feeling better. For those allergic to penicillin/amoxicillin there are several alternatives such as Keflex or Zithromax.

Strep throat is contagious but not as much as the common cold. The best way to avoid either condition is to wash your hands regularly, avoid touching your eyes and mouth, and keep a distance from those who are coughing or sneezing.

To alleviate the symptoms of a sore throat, I recommend the following:

- Take either acetaminophen (Tylenol), ibuprofen (Advil), or naproxen (Aleve).
- Gargle with warm salt water (1 teaspoon of salt per 6-8 oz. glass of water).
- Suck on throat lozenges, such as Chloraseptic or Cepacol.
- Suck on a flavored frozen treat, such as popsicles or just plain ice cubes.

# Swimmer's Ear

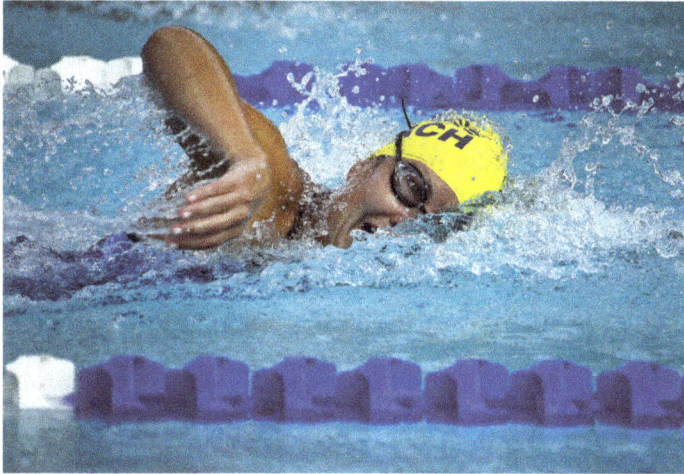

For what seems to be a minor health problem, swimmer's ear results in nearly 2.4 million doctor visits annually, and costs our health care system $500 million a year.

Swimmer's ear is an inflammation of the ear canal resulting from water entering the ear through swimming or bathing. This wet environment in the ear canal allows germs to multiply, thus leading to the painful infection. Warm temperatures, high humidity and more time spent in the water, increase the risk of acquiring swimmer's ear. That's why this malady peaks during the summer swimming season, occurring more frequently during the months of June, July, and August.

Symptoms of swimmer's ear include pain, tenderness, redness, and swelling of the ear canal. Occasionally there is a discharge from the ear. Other than being a very painful condition, swimmer's ear will almost always clear up completely leaving no long term side effects, such as chronic pain or hearing loss. This infection is treated with a course of antibiotic ear drops for about one week.

My recommendations to prevent swimmer's ear are:

- Avoid using Q tips, which can cause microtrauma to the ear canal thus making it more susceptible to infection.

- Dry ears as thoroughly as possible after water exposure.

- You can purchase commercial ear drops, available from pharmacies, to use in your ear after swimming to help prevent infection. As an alternative, a homemade solution can be used in place of the commercial one, by mixing 1 part rubbing alcohol to 1 part white vinegar, and placing several drops in the ear canal after water exposure. The alcohol helps to dry the ear, and the vinegar helps to keep germs from growing. Those with ear tubes or a possible hole in the ear drum should not put any type of drops in their ears.

More often than not, once an infection settles in the ear canal and the pain becomes nearly unbearable, a visit to the doctor may be necessary for prescription antibiotic ear drops.

## Adult Health Issues

I would like to discuss several important potentially lifesaving health issues for adults.

Women need Pap Smears to detect cancer of the cervix, which affects up to 12,000 women a year in the U.S. Women aged 21-29 should have a Pap test done every 3 years. Women 30-65 years should have a Pap test and an HPV test every 5 years. These are general recommendations that seem to change with time. Talk to your provider about what guidelines he or she would like to use.

Women also need to examine their breasts to detect breast cancer, which is the second leading cause of death in women, affecting almost 300,000 women annually. Self breast exams should be done monthly, beginning about age 20. Talk to your doctor about how to check your breasts, and have him or her check your breasts every 1-2 years. Also, mammogram recommendations seem to keep changing, so I recommend following your doctor's advice as to what age to begin, how often to have the test done, and how long to continue.

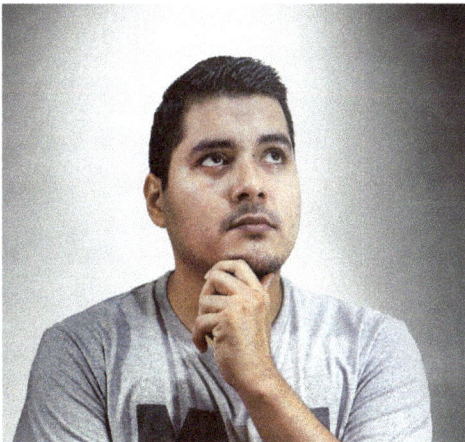

Men need to be concerned about prostate cancer. This disease affects up to 235,000 men yearly and is fatal to 28,000. There is an old saying in medicine that if a man lives long enough he will develop prostate cancer. Be aware that older men, Afro-American men, and men with a family history of prostate cancer are at a higher risk. Discuss with your doctor when screening with a PSA blood test and digital rectal exam should be begin and how often it need be done.

Lastly, both men and women need to be screened for colon cancer, another leading cause of death. About 150,000 cases are reported per year. Colon cancer is rarely seen before age 40. Colonoscopy has become exceedingly popular as the recommended diagnostic tool for the detection of colon cancer, and is recommended to be done beginning at age 50, and repeated every 7-10 years.

All the above recommendations have been general guidelines.  If you have a family history of a particular disease or other known risk factors, consult with your doctor. I have seen many lives saved by those who are willing to follow these  precautionary steps.

# Brain Health

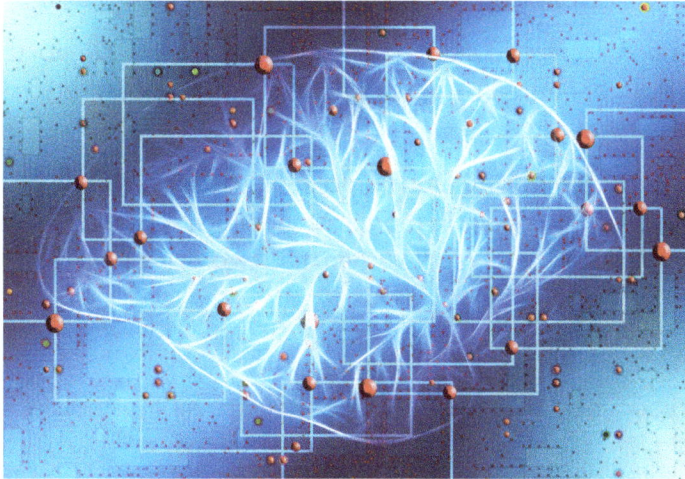

Throughout the general media, much is being said these days about improving and maintaining good health. Most of this information tends to emphasize our physical health, such as preventing conditions like diabetes, cardiovascular disease, cancer, arthritis etc. There is much less, but equally important information about keeping our brains healthy, especially as we age. Although current literature about maintaining brain health is geared toward the elderly population, what I am about to write is important for the entire population. No one is too young to start thinking about keeping their brains as healthy as possible.

The following are suggestions that anyone should follow to promote a healthy brain:

- Maintain a healthy cardiovascular system. This can be done by treating or preventing conditions, such as high blood pressure, high cholesterol, heart, and blood vessel disease.

- Exercise. Just 30 minutes of aerobic exercise at least 5 days a week will help to increase your heart rate and boost the delivery of oxygen and nutrients to the brain. (Even a small amount of exercise is better than none).

- Weight control. Try to maintain what your doctor figures should be your ideal weight to help avoid conditions, such as heart disease, diabetes, and overall stress and strain to the body.

- Watch your diet.  Try to eat more of what is referred to as the "Mediterranean diet." This diet avoids saturated and trans fats, and emphasizes lean meats, fruits, vegetables, fish, whole grains, and healthy fats, such as canola or olive oil, nuts, and legumes (beans or peas).

- Consider taking omega-3 supplements.  These are very important fatty acids which are very beneficial to the brain, and can be purchased at pharmacies and health food stores.

- Avoid unhealthy behaviors. Don't smoke or use any tobacco products, and if you choose to drink, do so in moderation, which is now considered to be no more than one drink a day for women and two drinks for men.

- Get adequate sleep.  Seven hours or more of good sleep is deemed necessary to maintain a healthy brain.

- Stimulate your mind. Challenge your brain with memory tasks, learn new information, engage in frequent social interactions, and pursue a variety of stimulating activities, such as crossword puzzles, sudoku, card games, etc.

- Don't worry, be happy. Think positively, learn to tolerate uncertainty, spend time with upbeat people, and try to improve your feelings of self worth.

Some people unfortunately will have abnormal deterioration of brain function due to bad genes, illness, or diseases over which they have no control. However, current research shows that the above mentioned suggestions could be very beneficial in maintaining a healthy brain.

# Exercise Benefits

The benefits of exercise are no longer theoretical. All recent studies concerning exercise and its effect on people, conclusively state that exercise will help most people live longer and healthier lives. Whether you are young or old, overweight or underweight, or even if you have a disability, exercise will benefit you.

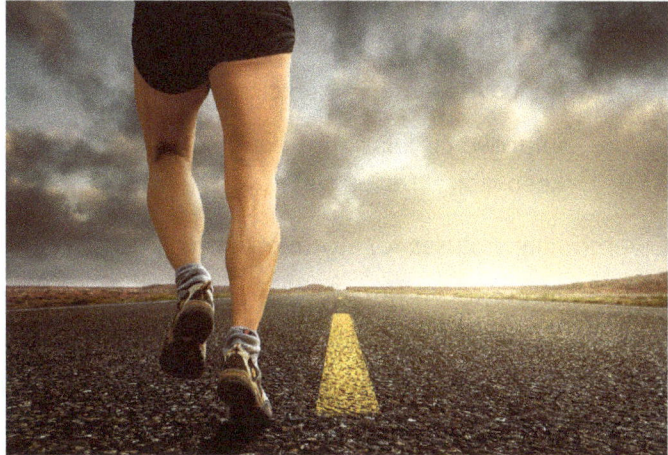

Most of us at any age wish we were more fit. Becoming older doesn't mean we have to become weaker and more fragile. Most physical changes of aging are due to inactivity and lifestyles that do not include regular exercise. Becoming and staying physically fit is the most important thing we can do to maintain our ability to continue doing the activities we now enjoy. The more fit one is, the more independent one may remain, as well as being happier and more satisfied with life.

It's truly never too late to begin a fitness program of regular exercise. I would like to list the beneficial reasons of exercising, and also give valid reasons for not putting it off any longer.

Reasons to exercise:

- Live longer.  Those who exercise regularly have been proven to add years to their lives.

- Help to lose weight.  Combined with proper diet, one will lose weight.

- Strengthen your heart. A stronger heart pumps blood more efficiently and doesn't have to beat as fast.

- Lift your mood.  People who exercise tend to be happier and less depressed.

- Improve chronic conditions. Exercise has been found to lower blood pressure and to improve diabetes and arthritis.

- Defend against illness. Exercise can boost the immune system and help fight off illness, especially flu and colds.

- Improve stamina. Exercise can provide more pep, energy, and less fatigue.

- Improve circulation. Exercise can improve our blood cholesterol and help keep our arteries clear.

Overcoming excuses for not exercising:

- Not enough time. Wake up earlier. Do several shorter periods of exercise throughout the day. Drive less, walk more.

- Tried it before didn't work. Set realistic goals. Pace yourself. Reinforce in your mind the benefits of exercise.

- I might injure myself by exercising. Start with a beginning exercise group. Pace yourself. Consider working with a trainer.

- It's too expensive. Joining a gym or having expensive equipment at home would be nice, but are not necessary. Watch an exercise video at home. Try just walking or climbing stairs.

- I'm not athletic. Most people are not particularly athletic. It is not a prerequisite for routine exercise. Anyone can and should exercise.

- It's just too much work. If exercise is just too much to do for your own good, then do it for those who love you. They will have you around longer, and will enjoy your health and happiness.

# Stress and Health

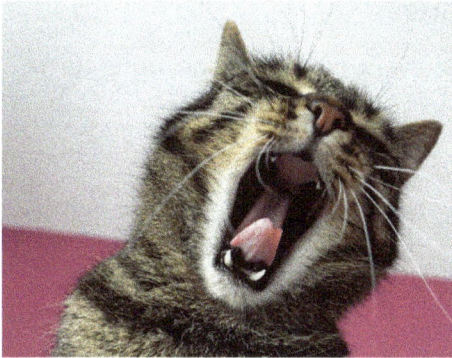

When we feel stressed, our bodies respond by releasing energy producing hormones, such as adrenaline and cortisol. This causes the "flight or fight" response, which physically prepares us to respond to a stressful situation. Have you ever had your heart pound quickly with rapid breathing when you've been suddenly startled by something, or when you've been in a very emotional argument? These reactions are caused by the "flight or fight" response.

Usually when the stress is over, the stress hormones revert back to normal levels, we feel better, and no harm done. If stress persists, and we are constantly bombarded by the stress hormones, many of our bodily functions can be disrupted leading to significant health problems.

Some of the health problems caused by chronic stress are:

- Heart disease, especially high blood pressure, heart attacks, and strokes
- Insomnia and depression
- Obesity and digestive problems
- Asthma and diabetes
- Alzheimer's disease and accelerated aging

Although we may not be able to eliminate all of our stresses, we can change how we respond to them. Stress management is a recognized method of dealing with stress by utilizing these strategies while in the throes of a stressful situation:

- Take some deep slow breaths and attempt to relax tensed up muscles, such as in the jaw and shoulders
- Reframe your stressful situation by attempting to find something positive

about what is going on at the time

- Focus on the present moment since much of our stress comes from something in the past or in our immediate future
- Keep things in perspective; does the stressful event really have any long term consequences?
- Think about all the good positive things in your life

Consider more long term techniques for dealing with life's stresses, such as:

- Regular exercise.
- Maintain a healthy diet and get adequate sleep/rest.
- Foster healthy, enjoyable friendships and have a good sense of humor.
- Practice yoga or other known relaxation techniques, and/or rely on your own personal religious beliefs to find peace and comfort.

Managing stress will not only improve our piece of mind, but will promote a healthier and longer life.

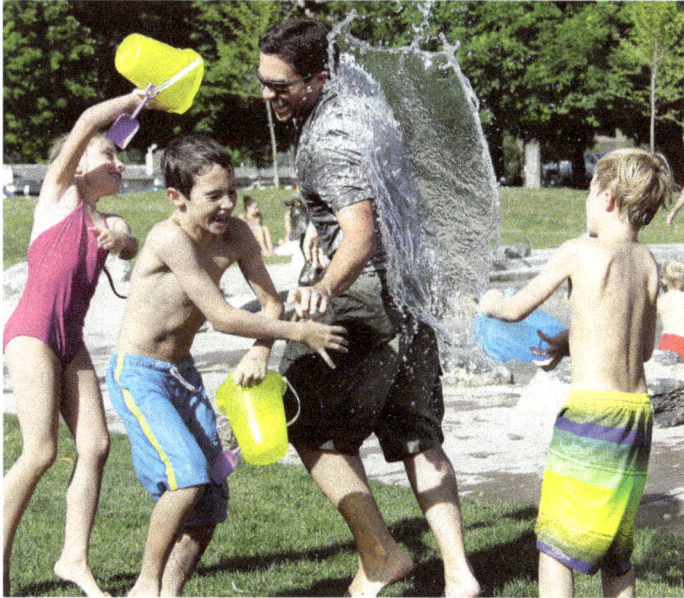

I'd like to talk about several common activities involving our children and how to ensure safety in order to avoid unnecessary injury.

Playground injuries, mostly from falls, account for over 200,000 emergency room visits per year. The highest risk group is 5-9 years of age. Young children need close adult supervision. Make sure that underneath the equipment there is an adequate shock absorbing material, such as chipped wood or any type of rubber product. Also, the equipment needs to be inspected to ensure that it appears to be in good repair.

Bicycling (300,000 emergency visits a year) and skateboarding (30,000 visits) are the leading cause of head injury accidents in children. Proper safety for these activities includes adult supervision of the younger children, routine bicycle maintenance, and mandatory use of head protective helmets. These helmets must be proper to the activity, and they must fit appropriately. But most importantly they must be worn!

Swimming accidents leading to drowning, are the second leading cause of injury death among children 14 years and younger. All pools must be adequately fenced in and have properly functioning gates. Injury can be avoided by not running around the pool, not jumping onto floating objects, and proper use of a diving board. Again, adult supervision is paramount in preventing swim related activities.

In 1971, trampoline injuries lead to the NCAA eliminating the trampoline from sports competition. I'm sure it's also why we don't see this event in the Olympics. Trampoline injuries cause 80,000 emergency visits per year for children age 5 and younger. If you own a trampoline, do not allow a smaller child to be on a trampoline with a larger child, as the smaller one is much more likely to be injured. One should follow the manufacturer's recommendations and not allow more than one person on a trampoline at a time. Safety netting around the trampoline is essential to protect a child, but is not fool-proof to prevent injuries. As with all the above activities, adult supervision is mandatory.

# Travel Health

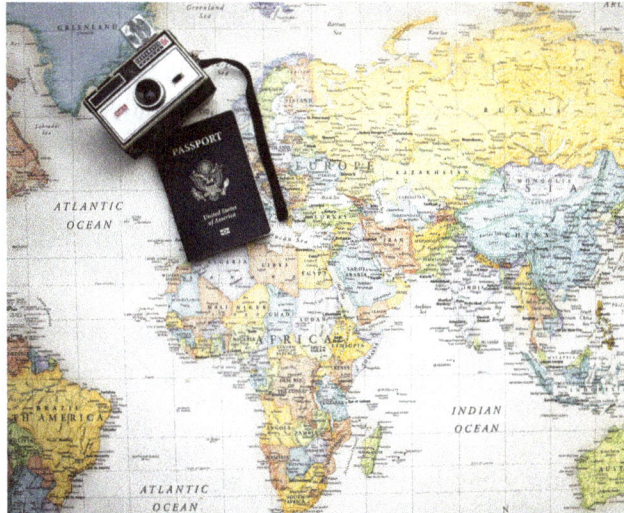

Traveling soon? Here's some travel advice.

First of all be prepared before you travel:

- Educate yourself about your destination; what will the weather be like? How are the sanitary conditions? Are there any safety or security issues? Will you need an electrical plug adapter?

- Visit your doctor before you leave if you have any health concerns or chronic medical conditions. Make this visit at least 5-6 weeks ahead of time as you might need immunizations.

- Make sure you have an adequate supply of your medications and pack them in a carry on rather than in luggage.

- Bring along a list of all your current medications, allergies, and blood type.

Important issues while traveling include:

- Prevent blood clots associated with prolonged sitting, by exercising your calf muscles while seated and/or get up and walk around every couple of hours.

- Minimize jet lag by staying well hydrated, avoiding alcohol and caffeine. Get plenty of rest prior to departing and upon arrival to your destination, adjust to the local schedule as fast as possible, and expose yourself to bright lights at the same time of day as before departure.

- Prevent traveler's diarrhea by washing hands frequently, avoiding precooked food such as buffets, street vendor food, and any water that is not bottled from a reputable source. Your doctor may want to prescribe antibiotics to take with you in case you come down with diarrhea.

- Motion sickness can be lessened by focusing on the horizon and not reading. Sit in the back of the vehicle and don't ride facing the rear.

- Avoid sunburn by bringing enough of an appropriate sunscreen and limiting time in sun, especially the first few days.

Do not travel if:

- You have recently had heart attack or stroke

- You have had recent surgery

- You have significant respiratory disease such as asthma or emphysema

- You have had recent injury to any vital organs

- You are ill with a bad cough, vomiting, diarrhea, or a fever of 100 degrees or above

Take along a travel health kit to include those things you commonly use at home for symptoms of illness or injury.

Do your best to deal with often encountered misfortunes such as missed flights, lost luggage, bad weather, disappointing accommodations, etc. You have no control over most of these things and allowing yourself to get stressed out can only make you feel more miserable. Look beyond these situations and imagine the joy that you will experience during your trip. Bon Voyage!

## Atrial Fibrillation

Atrial fibrillation is an irregular often rapid heart rate, causing the heart's two upper chambers to quiver instead of beating regularly. Fortunately, the lower two chambers still work normally and are able to pump the blood out of the heart, although not as efficiently. It is this inefficient pumping that can cause the frequent symptoms of palpitations, shortness of breath, weakness, and lightheadedness.

Atrial fibrillation is the most common heart arrhythmia. It is found in over 6 million Americans. It occurs in about 1% of individuals in their 60s increasing to up to 12% of adults in their 80s. Some 30% of people with atrial fibrillation are unaware of their condition.

Atrial fibrillation can be brought on by increasing age, prior coexisting heart disease, high blood pressure, thyroid disease, and drinking alcohol. It can come and go or it can be chronic and permanent. It is usually not life threatening, but it is a serious condition and needs to be treated.

There are two main goals in the treatment of atrial fibrillation. First is to attempt to control the rhythm, that is, get the rhythm back to the normal beating pattern. If a normal rhythm cannot be obtained then the second goal is to control the heart rate. Ideally one would want to have the rate 80 beats per minute or less. Both of these goals can be accomplished with medication.

If one is very symptomatic or has relatively new onset atrial fibrillation, the heart can be electrically treated with a small electrical shock while under brief anesthesia. However, this is rarely a permanent solution.

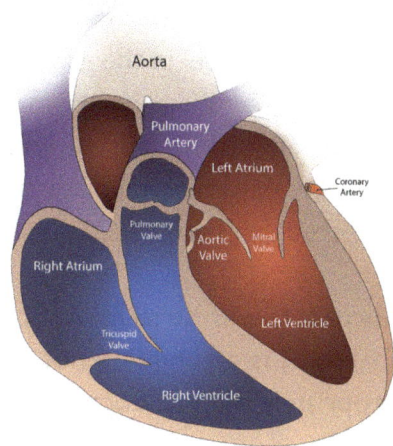

One of the  main problems with atrial fibrillation is the chance of having a stroke. Blood clots can form in the quivering upper chambers. If a clot breaks loose it can go to the brain causing a stoke. This can be prevented by taking a blood thinning medication. Another complication is heart failure due to a weakening of the heart muscle.

There is a new advanced procedure called ablation. In this case a catheter is inserted in a large blood vessel in the groin and threaded up into the heart. Through highly techni-cal computerized imaging, the trigger area for the fibrillation in the upper chamber is identified and lightly treated with high frequency radio waves. This destroys the area where the abnormal impulses of atrial fibrillation are generated. The success rate for this procedure is around 70% initially and up to 90% if a second procedure is necessary.

Many people with atrial fibrillation are living relatively normal lives today when properly managed. It is a condition not to be feared, but to be monitored closely and treated appropriately by your doctor.

# Cholesterol

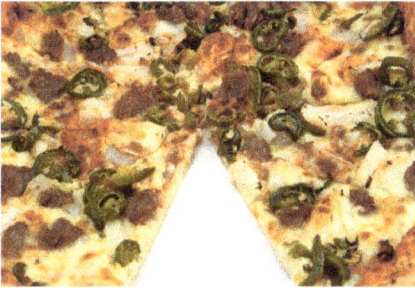

Cholesterol is a natural wax-like substance circulating through our blood vessels that helps to create healthy cells and hormones. A certain amount of cholesterol is definitely good for us, but an excess amount can cause fatty deposits in the lining of blood vessels. This makes it harder for blood to flow through the blood vessels bringing life sustaining oxygen, and may lead to either a heart attack or a stroke.

High cholesterol per se, has no symptoms and can only be detected by a blood test. One should have a baseline cholesterol blood test at age 35 for men, age 45 for women, and again every 5 years thereafter, or sooner if your doctor so determines because of your risk factors. Even children should be tested if they are obese, have high blood pressure, diabetes, or have a strong family history of high cholesterol.

Most of the cholesterol in our bodies is manufactured by our liver. A lesser amount comes from certain foods such as fatty meats, dairy products, and eggs. Therefore, a high cholesterol count can be due to either heredity or diet.

Cholesterol is carried through the blood attached to certain proteins. This combination of cholesterol and protein is called a lipoprotein, of which there are 3 types:

- Low density lipoproteins (LDL). Referred to as "bad cholesterol." These are the ones that cause the damage to blood vessels.

- Very low density lipoproteins (VLDL). These carry another type of fat called triglycerides which can also damage blood vessels.

- High density lipoproteins (HDL). Referred to as "good cholesterol." These actually pick up excess cholesterol and take it back to the liver.

Risk factors for developing high levels of cholesterol are smoking, diabetes, obesity, poor diet, lack of exercise, or a family history of heart disease.

The first thing to do for high cholesterol is to change one's lifestyle with emphasis on exercising and eating a healthy diet. If this doesn't work and your total cholesterol, particularly the LDL cholesterol remains high, your doctor will probably recommend medication. The actual choice of medication depends on several factors, such as your age, your current state of health, and possible side effects.

There are a variety of medications which help to lower cholesterol and triglycerides. They all do their work differently and have specific side effects. This is where your doctor will have to "fine tune" the medications to your specific needs and set up regular visits to monitor your progress.

The bottom line is to have your cholesterol checked and get it lowered to a more normal level. The results are in on this one; lowering an elevated cholesterol level will help to promote a longer and healthier life.

# Hypertension (High Blood Pressure)

High blood pressure, also known as hypertension, occurs when blood moves through our blood vessels at a greater than normal pressure, putting a strain on the heart. High blood pressure usually takes many years to develop and is said to affect 1 out of 3 adult Americans. It is easily detected and usually easily treated.

Normal blood pressure is 120/80. The upper number is called the systolic blood pressure and measures the pressure in your blood vessels when the heart beats. The lower number is called diastolic and measures the pressure in your blood vessels between beats when the heart relaxes. The higher the number means the greater the pressure your heart needs to pump the blood. High blood pressure for most adults usually necessitating medical treatment is defined as 140/90 or higher, and as new guidelines have suggested for those over 60 years of age, 150/90 or higher.

The most common type of high blood pressure is called primary hypertension and has no known cause. The less common type is called secondary hypertension because it is usually caused by something, such as kidney abnormalities, congenital heart defects, certain medications, and recreational drugs.

Blood pressure should be checked in children during their well child exams beginning at age three and every 1-2 years thereafter. If one has a family history of hypertension and especially as one gets older, blood pressure should be checked more often.

Many local pharmacies offer on site blood pressure machines for your convenience; however, it is preferable for the sake of accuracy and consistency to have your doctor check your blood pressure. Some people suffer from "white coat hypertension," which is a falsely elevated blood pressure in the doctor's office brought on by anxiety. These people, and others who so desire, can measure their blood pressure at home with the use of a blood pressure monitor, which can be purchased from most pharmacies.

When checking your blood pressure at home, remain seated with legs uncrossed for several minutes and avoid caffeine, alcohol, and exercise for at least 30 minutes prior to taking your blood pressure.

Some people with high blood pressure have no symptoms while others may have headaches, dizziness, or nosebleeds.

Risk factors for high blood pressure include increasing age, family history, and race. Women are more likely to develop hypertension after menopause.

Complications of high blood pressure include heart attack, heart failure, stroke, kidney, and eye disease. When symptoms of hypertension are addressed in a timely and properly treated, these complications occur much less frequently.

Life style changes can help to control and prevent high blood pressure.  Here's what you can do:

- Eat healthy foods such as fruits, vegetables, whole grains, and less saturated fat
- Lose weight if you are overweight
- Limit salt intake
- Limit alcohol.  If you drink, do so in moderation
- Don't smoke
- Participate in regular physical activity
- Manage stress

Controlling your blood pressure will go a long way to insure a longer and healthier life.

# CPR (Cardio-Pulmonary Resuscitation)

What would you do if you saw someone collapse and fall to the ground in front of you? Some might panic and do nothing, some might at least call for help, and others might attempt some form of CPR. There's good news for both the person who has collapsed as well as the bystander who needs to help out. The rules of CPR have changed and it can't become any simpler.

In the recent past we were advised to do mouth-to-mouth breathing as well as chest compressions. I think that many were confused as to how often to do the breathing and how fast to do the chest compressions. I've known many people who rightfully were hesitant to do mouth-to-mouth resuscitation on a stranger, and I think this very fact kept people from getting involved in the first place. It has been reported that only one third of those who suffer a cardiac arrest receive CPR from a bystander, and without CPR there is no chance of survival.

New research confirms that for bystanders without training, doing only chest compressions on adults is enough to restore life. It is now known that continuous uninterrupted chest compressions will deliver sufficient oxygen to the heart and brain, eliminating the need for mouth-to-mouth breathing. By making CPR easier, more lives have the potential to be saved.

A person who goes into cardiac arrest has usually gone into a heart rhythm call ventricular fibrillation. This means that the heart beats so fast and irregularly that the heart becomes totally ineffective, cannot pump blood, and therefore the body is completely deprived of oxygen. Without circulating oxygen a person cannot survive more than 7 or 8 minutes. In these crucial minutes if a heart is given an electrical shock by trained medical personnel, it has a chance of being changed back to a regular rhythm, thus restoring the oxygen flow to the body.

So, to answer my opening question, here's what to do when you see someone collapse and is unconscious and not breathing: first of all, when at all possible, call 911 to initiate an emergency medical response. Then, immediately begin to do chest compressions. Press with both hands on the center of the breastbone and press down hard approximately 100 times a minute. Do not stop until emergency medical personnel arrive or until you are too exhausted to continue.

I recently read in the local paper about a 50 year old bicyclist who collapsed from a cardiac arrest. A bystander who witnessed the event was willing to perform CPR, and the victim survived and is currently doing well. I believe that the victim, his wife and his children are happy that someone was willing to perform CPR on him.

Just think how meaningful it would be to save the life of a stranger, much less that of a loved one.

# Cardiovascular Issues in Women

Cardiovascular disease is the leading cause of death in women, responsible for more deaths each year than from all other causes combined. Between the ages of 45 to 65, one in nine women develops some form of cardiovascular disease. After age 65 the ratio climbs to one in three women.

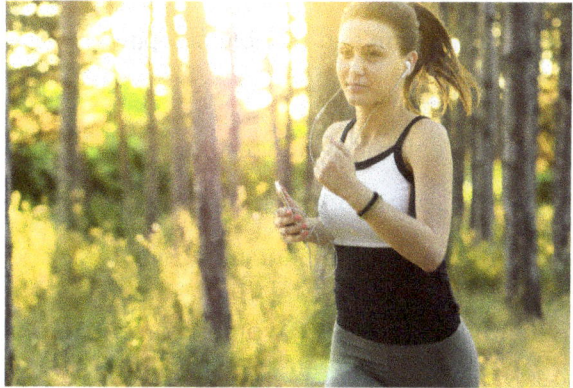

In a recent study, 58% of women 55 or younger hospitalized for a heart attack didn't suspect heart problems, despite having chest pain. Delayed treatment is one reason women are more likely to die after a heart attack than are men.

The following are risk factors for women that should be discussed with your doctor:

- Prior history of heart disease
- Age over 55
- Family history of early heart disease
- Diabetes
- Smoking
- High blood pressure
- Elevated cholesterol/triglycerides

Obesity has been associated with increased cardiac mortality and weight loss is beneficial, but repeated weight loss and weight gain, called "weight cycling," actually increases mortality. This is one of many reasons to lose weight and keep it off.

Common symptoms of heart attacks are chest pain often radiating to the left neck, jaw and shoulder, shortness of breath, nausea, and sweating. Women having a heart attack may have the above symptoms as well as the following:

- Fatigue and trouble sleeping

- Indigestion

- Feelings of anxiety

- Discomfort between the shoulder blades

- Sense of impending doom

Recommendations for women to reduce cardiovascular disease:

- Daily physical exercise

- Avoid cigarette smoking

- Weight reduction

- Healthy diet

- Treatment of high blood pressure, diabetes, and high cholesterol

If you have any of the above issues, I recommend that you work closely with your doctor to achieve a longer and healthier life.

# Heart Health

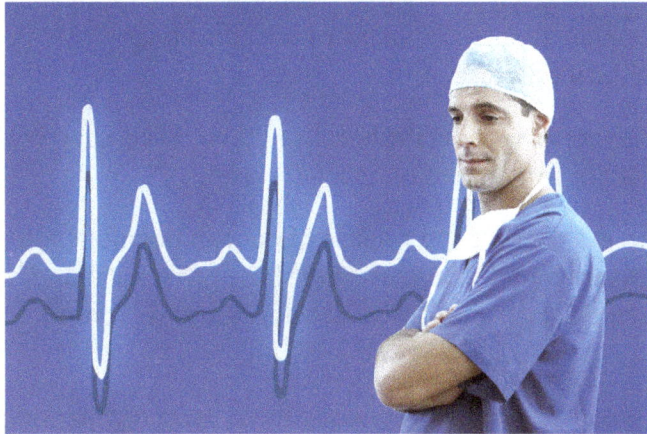

You don't have to spend a lot of money or take medication to maintain a healthy heart, just follow these guidelines:

1. Quit smoking. Smoking causes high blood pressure, decreases exercise tolerance, increases blood clotting, and doubles the odds of a heart attack.

2. If you drink alcohol, do so in moderation. Alcohol can increase the blood pressure and in higher doses can significantly weaken heart muscle.

3. Exercise the heart as much as you would do for any other muscle to help strengthen it and keep it healthy. 30 minutes a day of moderate intensity exercise, such as brisk walking five days a week, or 20 minutes of vigorous activity, such as jogging three days a week. Try to make your exercise enjoyable (bring a friend or listen to music) and be persistent.

4. Eat plenty of fiber, such as fruits, nuts, whole grains, and vegetables. Avoid saturated fats, for example those found in most meats, chicken skin, and many dairy products. Instead, eat good fats, such as olive oil, nuts, avocados, and olives.

5. Maintain a normal blood pressure. High blood pressure increases the work load on the heart and eventually will cause it to become thicker, stiffer, and weaker, which can lead to heart attacks and heart failure.

6.  Maintain as normal a weight as possible.  As with hypertension, excess weight also increases the workload of the heart leading to the same end result of heart damage. Recent research shows that people who carry most of their weight around their middle (apple shaped as opposed to pear shaped), are at an even greater risk of heart disease.

7.  Controlling diabetes is important because up to three quarters of people with diabetes will die of some form of heart disease.

8.  Keep calm.  Stress triggers the release of certain hormones that have an adverse effect on the heart muscle. Studies have shown that calm and happy people have fewer heart attacks than those who are angry and discontent. "Don't worry – be happy."

9.  Avoid salt as much as possible especially if you have high blood pressure. The recommended daily limit of salt is 2,300 mg. (one teaspoon). Try to avoid processed food and read food labels to steer clear of the worst offenders.

10. Maintain adequate levels of vitamin D. Research shows that people with low levels of vitamin D were twice as likely to have a heart attack. Follow your doctor's advice as to proper dosage.

The above guidelines are tried and true methods of significantly improving your odds of decreasing heart disease and thereby promoting a healthier, happier, and longer life.

Heart attacks are the leading cause of adult deaths in the U.S. causing over one million deaths a year. Today, thanks to better awareness on the part of the public and improved treatments, most people who have a heart attack now survive. Treatment needs to begin within one hour of the beginning of symptoms. Therefore, if you or someone you know may be having a heart attack, call 911 immediately to be transported to the nearest hospital emergency room.

A heart attack occurs when blood flow to a section of the heart becomes blocked. This deprives the heart muscle of oxygen and can cause that section of the muscle to die.

The coronary arteries are the blood vessels that bring oxygen-rich blood to the heart muscle. Over a period of time, one or more of these arteries can become narrowed due to a build up of cholesterol, which is called a *plaque*. When a plaque ruptures, a blood clot can form in the blood vessel and blocks the flow of blood to the heart muscle. This is what usually causes a heart attack. The severe consequences of a heart attack include heart failure and life threatening arrhythmia (irregular heartbeat). Heart failure is when the heart muscles are too damaged and weak to adequately pump blood through our bodies. This condition usually takes its toll sometime after the heart attack.

The most common threat to life from a heart attack is an arrhythmia called ventricular fibrillation, which causes the heart to beat so irregularly that it cannot pump blood at all. When someone dies immediately of a heart attack (cardiac arrest) it is usually from ventricular fibrillation. If a person in ventricular fibrillation is given an electrical shock with a defibrillator within the first 5-6 minutes after a cardiac arrest, a normal rhythm can occasionally be restored thus saving one's life. This is why timely emergency response is critical to the survival of a victim of cardiac arrest. Most of our communities have fire department EMTs and paramedics who will usually respond first to a 911 call and are trained to begin potential life saving treatment.

Heart attack risk factors include:

1.  High blood pressure
2.  High cholesterol levels
3.  Cigarette smoking
4.  Obesity
5.  Lack of physical activity
6.  Diabetes
7.  Family history of heart attack
8.  Male gender
9.  Over indulgence of alcohol

Typical signs and symptoms of a heart attack include:

1.  Chest pain usually described as a pressure sensation in the middle of the chest which may be mild or severe.  This pain is often mistaken as heartburn or indigestion, and can radiate to the jaw, neck, or arm, usually on the left side.

2.  Shortness of breath.

3.  Nausea, lightheadedness, and/or breaking into a cold sweat.

Don't "tough out" the symptoms of a heart attack. Within minutes of heart attack symptoms one should call 911. Being attended to as soon as possible by trained paramedics is paramount for increased chance of survival. If there is no access to emergency medical services, which is rare in our communities, have someone drive you immediately to a hospital emergency room and preferably not to your doctor's office, clinic, or urgent care center. Try not to drive yourself, as you may be putting yourself or others in danger if your condition worsens.

Limiting risk factors and understanding the symptoms of a heart attack and seeking timely emergency medical care, will go a long way in helping people survive heart attacks and live full active lives.

# Heart Attack Part 2

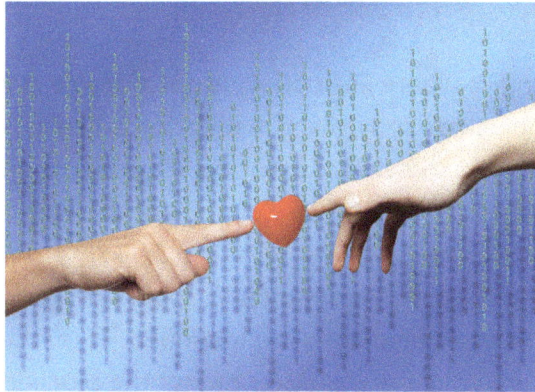

## EMERGENCY TREATMENT

It is important to know that when a heart attack strikes, "time equals muscle." The longer the delay in seeking medical care the more heart muscle will be damaged. I'd like to talk about what happens to a person after suffering a non-fatal heart attack. A person with chest pain arriving to the emergency room is immediately placed on a cardiac monitor to measure heart rhythm. Vital signs are taken with blood pressure and pulse being of primary importance. Oxygen is administered and an aspirin tablet is given. An EKG (electrocardiogram) is done and blood is drawn and sent to the laboratory. An IV will be started to allow for the immediate treatment of any necessary drugs. The EKG will verify the heart rhythm and rate, as well as demonstrating any possible damage to the heart muscle. Both the EKG and blood tests may be repeated over a period of time to check for any ongoing changes.

When the diagnosis is confirmed, and when the patient is in stable condition, he or she may immediately undergo coronary angiography, which is a special X-ray of the heart and blood vessels. It can identify the location of the blockages in the coronary arteries. This exam is performed by a medical specialist who passes a thin flexible tube called a catheter through an artery in either an arm or the groin. A dye is injected through the catheter and as it passes through the coronary arteries, it is seen on the X-ray and localizes the blockage. With the blockage located, the doctor can then open the blockage (angioplasty) and restore the blood flow. Sometimes a small mesh tube called a stent can be placed in an attempt to keep the blockage open.

In some smaller communities where angioplasty is not available, another method of opening the coronary artery blockage is by giving medication called a thrombolytic, commonly called a "clot buster," which can help to dissolve a clot. The sooner after a heart attack this is done the better for survival with less damage of the heart muscle.

In some cases, doctors may perform emergency bypass surgery at the time of a heart attack especially when multiple blockages are identified. This procedure involves sewing another blood vessel from your own body to bypass the blocked coronary artery, thus restoring blood flow to the heart.

Most people can return to work and the activities they enjoy after having a heart attack. Exercise has many benefits for people after a heart attack. It can strengthen the heart muscles as well as making one feel more energetic. The amount of activity you can do depends on the condition of your heart. Your doctor can help you plan the necessary steps for your recovery.

# Palpitations

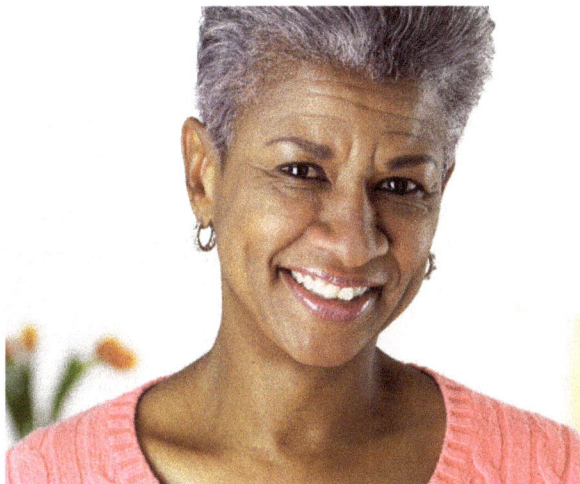

Patients who come to a doctor complaining of palpitations are usually worried they may have some serious problem with their heart. They often describe the feeling that their hearts are "flip-flopping," missing a beat, beating faster, or beating irregularly. Palpitations, whether harmless (as most of them are) or serious, should not be ignored. A medical evaluation is recommended, especially if one has palpitations associated with dizziness, shortness of breath, chest pain, or fainting.

Palpitations are usually caused by the heart beating prematurely (too soon) before the next normal beat occurs. When this happens, one feels the "flip-flop" sensation in their chest. Since the palpitation is only a skipped beat, the heart can still function normally, therefore usually not causing any health risk. In rare cases, however, palpitations may be a sign of a potentially serious heart problem that may require treatment.

Quite often a cause for palpitations is not found, but some known factors include:

- Strong emotional responses, such as anxiety, stress, or fear
- Caffeine, nicotine, and alcohol
- Strenuous exercise
- Taking cold and cough medications that contain the decongestant pseudoephedrine (Sudafed)

Serious complications of palpitations are:

- Fainting from a significant drop in blood pressure
- Stroke from causing lack of oxygen-rich blood to the brain
- Heart failure from the heart pumping ineffectively
- Cardiac arrest from a heart beating so irregularly that blood circulation stops

A medical evaluation for palpitations will usually involve a physical exam, blood tests, and an electrocardiogram (EKG). Your doctor may also order a portable heart monitor which may detect palpitations not found on the EKG.

The bottom line is that heart palpitations are usually more bothersome than they are serious, but check with your doctor just to be safe.

# Stroke

A stroke occurs when the blood supply to the brain is suddenly altered. This can occur from a clot in a blood vessel blocking blood flow to brain tissue, or less often from a burst blood vessel that can damage an area of the brain. These conditions cause brain cells to die or at least become damaged, which can cause temporary or permanent changes in body and mind function. Every year 800,000 Americans have a stroke.

A transient ischemic attack (TIA), also called a mini stroke, is a temporary stroke-like condition which usually resolves in a number of hours. TIAs are often a warning of a future more serious stroke and also need to be dealt with emergently.

If you, a loved one, or friend are having symptoms of a stroke or a TIA, do not go to your doctor's office or to an urgent care clinic. Be driven by a friend or family member immediately to a hospital emergency room, or call 911 and be taken by ambulance. Research shows that people who arrive at the hospital by ambulance get there quicker, get seen quicker, and are more likely to get necessary treatment in time to prevent permanent brain damage. Do not hesitate or delay. Don't worry about a "false alarm." Better safe than sorry.

Risk factors for a stroke include:

- Age – Most occur in older adults, but up to a quarter of them strike people younger than 65
- Family history – Especially if sibling or parent had stroke
- Gender – Men more than women; pregnant women are at higher risk
- High blood pressure, increased cholesterol, and smoking
- Diabetes and heart disease (especially atrial fibrillation)

Signs and symptoms of a stroke:

- Numbness or weakness of one side of face, arm, or leg
- Sudden difficulty speaking, remembering, or thinking
- Trouble with vision or swallowing
- Sudden difficulty walking or balancing
- Sudden severe headache

There is a clot busting medication which can stop most strokes in their tracks if given promptly enough. Guidelines call for this drug to be given within 4 1/2 hours after the very first sign of a stroke. If you think someone is having a stroke, the National Stroke Association recommends the F.A.S.T test:

- F  stands for face – Ask person to smile.  Does one side of face droop?
- A  stands for arm – Ask to raise both arms, does one drift downward?
- S  stands for speech – Is speech slurred?
- T  stands for time – Call 911. Get person to hospital A.S.A.P.

## Vaccinations

I recently tuned in to a local radio station talk show where the host and a "non-medical doctor" were criticizing vaccinations by citing false information and providing their personal bias. I would like to offer my view of vaccinations.

Most vaccines contain parts of a germ or toxin that have been made so weak that they can no longer cause illness, but will stimulate one's immune system to make antibodies against that specific disease. Therefore, in the future when one is exposed to that particular germ, the antibodies should prevent that person from getting sick.

Since vaccines were first developed in the late 1700's, millions of lives have been saved. Smallpox which wiped out entire civilizations has actually been totally eliminated from the face of the earth because of the smallpox vaccine. I watched friends come down with polio in the 1950's and become permanently paralyzed. This was a fearful disease until the polio vaccine banished it from the U.S.

We have effectively controlled outbreaks of common diseases such as measles, mumps, diphtheria, and chicken pox. Before the chicken pox vaccine became available, over 11,000 Americans were hospitalized and over 100 died each year from chicken pox. It is estimated that measles, one of the most contagious diseases in the world, could cause almost 3 million deaths worldwide if vaccinations were stopped.

Commonly asked questions: Are vaccines safe? I believe they are. Thousands of people take part in clinical trials before a vaccine is approved. Millions of people are vaccinated every year. Some people may get local reactions of pain, swelling, and redness at the vaccination site, but this lasts only a few days.

- Can vaccines cause autism? \I know this is an extremely controversial issue but there is no scientific evidence to directly link vaccine and autism. Common pediatric vaccines with the exception of some flu shots, no longer contain mercury or thimerosal, chemicals often implicated with vaccine side effects.

- Are infants getting too many shots at once?  In general, infants tolerate these vaccines very well. Every day infants come into contact with millions of bacteria, viruses and pollen which impact their immune systems. Delaying shots can leave a child unprotected against certain diseases, many of which can have dangerous complications such as seizures, brain damage, blindness, and even death.

- If everyone gets vaccinated, will my child still need them?  It is true that an unimmunized child has less of a chance of catching a disease if everyone else is immunized, but if a larger number of children are not immunized, then there will be a greater chance of highly contagious diseases spreading through the population.

- How long does immunity last after getting a vaccine?  Many vaccines, such as measles and hepatitis B, cause lifetime immunity.  Others, such as tetanus, last for many years, but require booster shots.

The bottom line is that vaccinations have saved millions of lives, significantly lessened, and in cases eliminated certain killer diseases, and have played a very significant role in the increased life span of humans over the past several generations. There are many well intentioned individuals and groups who advocate against vaccinations. I hear what they are saying, but scientific evidence and multiple studies have demonstrated the safety and effectiveness of vaccinations. Talk to your doctor about the vaccinations that you or your child may need.

# Routine Adult Immunizations

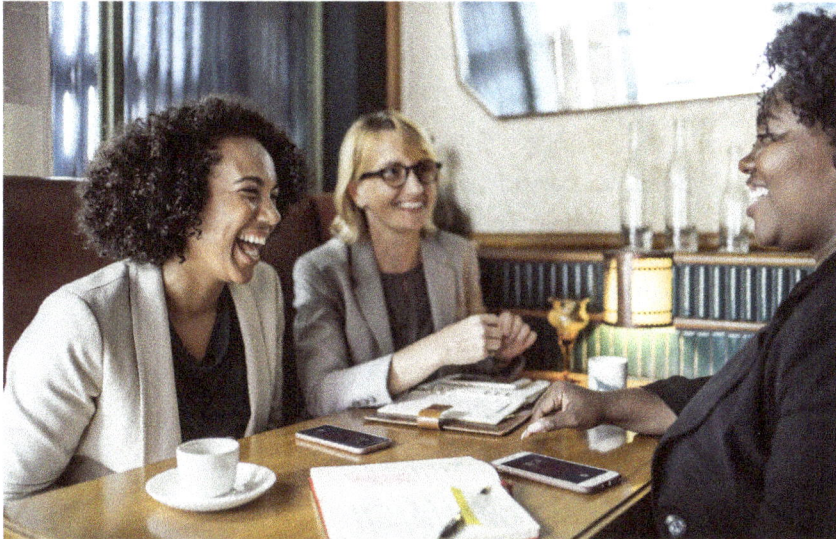

Immunizations for adults and children have been proven safe and are very effective in preventing many illnesses, as well as having saved a countless number of lives from potentially deadly diseases and epidemics.

Why do adults need immunizations? Some adults incorrectly assume that vaccines they received in childhood will protect them for the rest of their lives. This is mostly true, except that:

- Some adults believe they received vaccinations as a child, but never actually did

- Newer vaccines were not available previously

- Effectiveness of the vaccine lessens with time

- As we age, we become more susceptible to common infections, such as caused by influenza (flu) and pneumococcal disease (pneumonia)

These are what I feel are the most important adult vaccines:

- Influenza – Every fall season for all adults especially for those over 65 years of age

- Tetanus with diphtheria and pertussis (whooping cough), then tetanus and diphtheria every 10 years thereafter

- Pneumococcal (pneumonia) – for those 65 years or older. There are several types available, consult your doctor

- Shingles – everyone 60 years or older

- Rubella (German measles) – women of child-bearing age

Young women and men may want to check with their doctors about HPV (human papilloma virus). Travelers, especially those going to Africa, Latin America, or Asia, should consider hepatitis A and typhoid vaccines.

Next time you have a reason to see your doctor, talk about routine immunizations and make sure you are up to date. Remember, it pays to keep a step ahead of illness and disease.

# Childhood Immunizations

Small pox, polio, diphtheria, tetanus, measles, mumps, and rubella, are all potential life-threatening diseases that have been almost completely eliminated from our society during our lifetimes. The reason for this is because of the routine childhood immunization program that has been widely accepted in the United States, as well as most of the modern world.

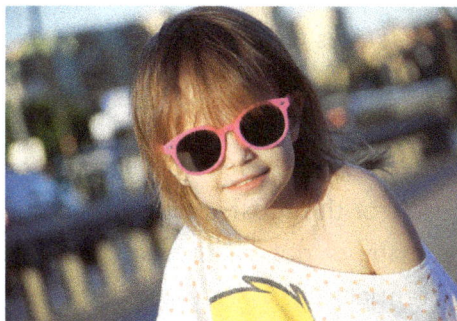

We often hear about the supposed side effects of immunizations, but we rarely hear about children getting the very diseases that the vaccines protect against. That's because the immunization program has worked so well in preventing diseases that could have killed millions and caused untold suffering. In fact, we've been so successful immunizing children and preventing diseases that some might wonder whether vaccines are still needed.

Here's why immunizations are still necessary:

- Newborn babies are immune to many diseases because they have antibody protection from the mothers. This immunity is mostly gone by the end of the first year of life leaving unvaccinated babies susceptible to the above mentioned vaccine-preventable illnesses.

- Although our country has virtually eliminated these diseases, many Third World countries with poor immunization programs are still plagued by vaccine-preventable illnesses. These diseases are only a plane ride away. An infected traveler could bring such an illness back to the states, where it could spread rapidly if people were not adequately immunized.

- In the U.S., pertussis (whooping cough) is making a comeback, and tetanus is still infecting some people. Widespread immunization is necessary because it helps to keep a disease from spreading within a population. This helps to protect those few who, whether by choice or necessity, are not immunized.

- Immunizations are safe. Many well controlled scientific studies have all concluded that there is no scientific or statistical relationship between immunizations and autism.

Many states (but not the federal government) are currently enacting laws for mandatory vaccinations in school age children.

Until vaccine preventable illnesses are eliminated worldwide, as with deadly smallpox (a result of the most successful immunization program ever), I strongly recommend that as many of our children as possible be routinely immunized and thus protected from potentially life threatening diseases.

# HPV – Human Papillomavirus

HPV, also known as *human papillomavirus*, is a sexually transmitted virus disease that will infect almost all men and women with at least one of the many types of known HPV strains at some point in their lifetime. The majority of people will never know they are infected because they will show no symptoms, and may unknowingly pass HPV through sexual activity to a partner. About 90 million Americans are currently infected with the virus and up to 20 million people become infected yearly. Fortunately, most of those with HPV never develop symptoms and 9 out of 10 infections resolve after several years.

HPV commonly causes warts in the genital areas as well as cancer. Both men and women can get cancer of the throat and mouth, as well as the anus and rectum. Women can also be affected by cancer of the vagina, vulva, and cervix, and men by cancer of the penis. At this time, men are affected more by HPV-related throat cancer than women are from cervical cancer.

HPV is transmitted by the variety of sex acts in which people indulge. HPV can be passed on to a partner even from someone not showing any symptoms, and is passed on through direct contact with an infected partner when the vulva, vagina, cervix, penis, or anus touches someone else's genitals, or mouth and throat during sex. HPV can also be passed on by a contaminated sex toy, but it cannot be passed on by toilet seats or other objects.

The good news in all of this is that there is now a vaccine to help prevent HPV. This vaccine is recommended prior to ever having sex. Therefore it is recommended to begin vaccinations for boys and girls around ages 11 to 12. It is given as a series of three shots. Teens who were not vaccinated when younger should still receive the vaccine. It is also recommended for young men through age 21 and for young women through age 26, regardless if they are sexually active or not.

HPV vaccines work extremely well. Studies have demonstrated nearly a 100 percent protection for many of the HPV cancers. There has been no evidence that HPV vaccine loses its effectiveness with time nor that it can actually cause the HPV infection. The three current vaccines available went through years of extensive testing before they were released and have been found to be extremely safe.

HPV vaccination is based on age, not sexual experience. Even though HPV is often transmitted during the first sexual encounters, the vaccine should still be given to those who qualify (as mentioned above) even after having had sex, as there are a number of HPV types that would still be prevented.

As with most vaccines, there are rare side effects to the vaccine including pain, redness, or swelling at the injection site, as well as headache, fatigue, nausea, and joint or muscle pain.

There is no test for men to detect HPV. For women, the test can be done at the same time as the Pap test. A Pap test plus an HPV test (co-testing) is the preferred way to detect early cervical cancers or pre-cancers in women 30 and older.

I know that there are those who are opposed to vaccines in general and that there are those who don't want to talk to their children about sex and its potential consequences. However, this is a very important and potentially serious health issue, and I would advise a parent to discuss HPV vaccination with their child's medical provider.

## Bladder Infections (Cystitis)

Acute cystitis is the medical term for a bladder infection, and is the most common cause of what is generally known as a urinary tract infection. It affects up to 10 million Americans a year, mostly women. About 40% of women at sometime during their lifetime will have a bladder infection, and many will have multiple episodes.

Risk factors include:

- Female gender:  This is the most common risk factor because the female urethra (the tube that connects the bladder to the outside of the body) is very short allowing germs an easier entrance to the bladder

- Sexual activity

- Use of a diaphragm

- Personal hygiene

Symptoms:

- A burning sensation when urinating

- Frequent urination often of small amounts

- A very strong urge to urinate

- Blood in the urine (scary but not necessarily serious)

- Strong odor or cloudy urine

If you experience any of the above symptoms regardless of your gender, see your doctor. If you do have an infection, you will prescribed an appropriate antibiotic

The most common germ identified is the E. coli germ, which is found in the human intestine. There are at least a half a dozen different antibiotics, which can be used to treat bladder infections. Fortunately, in most cases of acute cystitis only three days of treatment are necessary. You may also be prescribed a medication called phenazopyridine, which quickly improves the discomfort of a bladder infection. This is helpful before the antibiotic "kicks in." This drug, under the name of Uristat, can now be purchased over-the-counter, and can be useful to begin treating your symptoms before you get to see the doctor. Be aware that it will turn your urine a dark orange color.

Many people have the notion that drinking cranberry juice will help to cure a bladder infection. Cranberry juice does not help treat an active infection, it only helps prevent infections in those who get them frequently. Those who rely on cranberry juice to treat an infection are only delaying the proper treatment with an antibiotic. If a bladder infection goes untreated it may worsen and even spread to the kidneys, causing a more serious kidney infection.

Preventing bladder infections:
- Drink enough liquids to flush the bacteria out of the bladder
  (Drink more than you feel you really need to)
- Avoid a full bladder and empty the bladder whenever the urge is present
- Practice good hygiene. "Wipe from front to back." And wash the skin around the genital area daily.
- Change sanitary pads and tampons frequently
- Avoid bubble baths, which can irritate the urethra and mimic an infection

Fortunately, bladder infections are not usually serious if recognized and treated in time.

# Bronchitis

Acute bronchitis is an infection causing inflammation of the lung's airways, and is one of the most common of human ailments. It usually begins with head cold symptoms, such as a runny nose, sinus congestion, or a sore throat. It is almost always caused by a virus and rarely by bacteria. If a cough is not due to pneumonia, influenza, or asthma, it is most likely what we call bronchitis.

Most people actually feel fairly well with bronchitis, except for having a persistent nagging cough. Fever is rare and mucus production may or may not be present. A very common misperception is that colored mucus, especially green, indicates a bacterial infection and therefore the need for antibiotics. Recent scientific evidence supports that virus infections also produce green mucus.

Those who smoke are much more susceptible to bronchitis because of the damage done by the smoke to the lining of the breathing tubes of the lungs. This allows germs to enter the lungs more easily, causing an infection.

Many patients request antibiotics in hopes of quickly ridding themselves of the cough and therefore  visit their doctor as soon as symptoms begin, so that they may "nip it in the bud." Some think that antibiotics helped them on previous occasions, but there is no proven benefit for these drugs in the treatment of most cases bronchitis.  Inappropriate antibiotic use can cause unnecessary side effects, (diarrhea and yeast infections to mention a few), increase the cost of medical care, and lead to the development of resistant germs. This means that many of our commonly used antibiotics are no longer effective against many germs and there are very few new and extremely expensive antibiotics being developed.

Treatment for bronchitis is directed towards relieving the symptoms. For the head cold symptoms that come with bronchitis, an oral decongestant pill, such as Sudafed (pseudoephrine), as well as a decongestant nasal spray, such as Afrin (oxymetazoline hydrochloride), can be used to combat nasal and sinus congestion. Afrin spray works well to open up clogged nasal passages but should not be used for more than one week to avoid rebound (worsening) congestion. Tylenol (acetaminophen) or Advil (ibuprofen) can be used for the relief of aches and pains. Drinking plenty of liquids has proven to loosen and cause thinning of mucus.

For cough symptoms, over the counter cough medicines with dextromethorphan, such as Robitussin DM or Vicks 44 may be helpful. A recent study has recommended the use of a natural cough remedy using a mixture of 5 parts honey and one part instant coffee crystals. Take one tablespoon of the mixture in about 6 ounces of water every 6 hours for cough. Also, for a cough that makes the lungs feel tight or wheezy, a doctor may prescribe a brief course of an inhaled medication commonly used for asthmatics.

In summary, most coughs that we call bronchitis can last at least 2 to 3 weeks, are almost always caused by a virus, and antibiotic treatment is usually not helpful. However, if at any time you have a cough with a fever, you should see your doctor.

# Fever

Fever is defined as an elevation of body temperature, which normally is 98.6°F (37°C). Normal temperature can vary from 97.4°F (36.4°C) to 99.9°F (37.7°C). A fever is not an actual illness, but is a sign that the body is dealing with an infection. Some scientific evidence indicates that a moderate fever may actually be beneficial in helping the body to overcome an infection. There are also some very rare non infectious causes of fever, such as heat stroke or drug related fevers.

Temperature can be measured in several different ways. The most convenient, but unfortunately not the most accurate method, is using a special thermometer to measure ear drum temperature. For infants the most accurate method is a rectal temperature. Axillary (armpit) temperature is not as accurate. For adults, an oral temperature is easy to obtain and is accurate

When a fever begins and it is on the rise, a person feels chilled and may shiver. One tends to wrap one's self up in blankets and turn up the heat. When the body temperature reaches its new set point, one might feel quite hot, and as the fever begins to lower, may break into a sweat.

It is important to understand that a fever is not serious other than perhaps making one feel even more uncomfortable. A fever is not dangerous to the human body until it reaches 106°F (41°C) or even 107°F. (41.7°C) In my clinical experience, I have never dealt with a patient with that high of a fever and have never seen anyone suffer serious effects of a fever, although such cases are occasionally reported.

What's more important than just the level of a fever is to find what type of infection is causing it. In general, the higher the fever the more serious is the infection. When temperatures reach and remain 104°F (40°C) or above, serious infections such as pneumonia, kidney infections, or meningitis must be ruled out.

A rapid rise or fall in temperature may cause a fever induced seizure in a small number of children usually younger than 5 years of age. These events can be very frightening for the parents, but are usually of no harm to the child. Medical care should be sought immediately after such an occurrence.

It is usually not necessary to treat a fever of under 102°F (39°C). Treating a fever of 102°F or above will probably help one feel more comfortable. The mainstay of treatment is using either acetaminophen (Tylenol) or ibuprofen (Advil). There is no proof that one works better than the other.  A person with liver disease should avoid Tylenol and a person with stomach ulcers or kidney disease should avoid Advil. Either medication given in a proper dose according to the manufacturer's directions on the container and given regularly at every six hours should be effective. Quite often these two medications are given in alternating doses and although there is no scientific evidence of the effectiveness of this, many people swear by it. I don't have a problem with this method except that it can be confusing remembering which dose was given, and that it also increases the possibility of giving the wrong dose to a child.

Of equal importance for treating a fever is keeping a person cool by not bundling up with too much clothing or bed covering. A person who is sick with a fever needs less, not more covering. They will not get sicker; in fact, they will feel better. Drinking adequate liquids and/or sponge bathing in a tub of lukewarm water, is also important in fever control.

The following are recommendations as to when to seek medical advice/treatment for an illness with a fever:

1.  An infant younger than 3 months of age with a rectal temperature of 100.4°F (38°C) or higher

2.  A child 3-6 months of age with a temperature up to 102°F (38.9°C) and seems unusually irritable, uncomfortable, lethargic, or has a temperature higher than 102°F (38.9°C) regardless of symptoms

3.  A child older than 6 months with a temperature higher than 102°F (38.9°C) that lasts longer than one day but shows no other signs

4.  Any ill child who is very irritable, lethargic, or poorly responsive

5.  An adult with a temperature at any time of 104°F (40°C), or 101°F (38.3°C) or above, lasting for more than a few days

Consult with your doctor if you have any concerns about an illness with a fever.

# Lyme/Tick Disease

I'd like to discuss tick bite and signs and symptoms of Lyme disease.

Neither the tick's body nor its head burrows into the skin. Instead, the tick attaches by its mouthparts. It is said (but not conclusively proven) that an infected tick can transmit an infection only after it has been attached, taken blood from its host, and fed for 24 to 48 hours. If you find a tick on you that is unattached and non-engorged, it is also said to be unlikely to have transmitted an infection. Look carefully for the immature nymphal ticks, which are the size of a sesame seed, as they are the ones most likely to pass on the infection. It helps to shower after clearing brush or walking in wild lands to help clear off any non attached ticks from your body.

The proper method of removing a tick is to use a fine pair of tweezers and grasp the tick as close to the skin as possible. Pull it straight out, gently but firmly, without jerking or twisting. After removing the tick, wash your hands and the skin around the bite thoroughly with soap and water.

If, after removal, you see anything remaining in the skin, this represents tiny mouthparts of the tick. It is not the tick's "head" and it cannot increase the risk of transmission of Lyme disease once the tick body is removed. If you are unable to remove the mouth parts easily, as you would a splinter, leave it alone and the skin should eventually heal. If you are concerned see your doctor.

Quite often, after an obvious tick bite, a red rash may develop at the site of the bite within the first 24 to 48 hours. A rash that develops this quickly after the bite is usually an allergic or sensitivity reaction to the saliva of the tick. It rarely grows beyond 2 inches, needs no treatment, and disappears within a few days. This immediate type of rash is usually of no concern.

The actual Lyme's rash, called *erythema migrans*, is reported to occur in at least 50 percent of infected tick bites. It is described as a red rash that is usually neither itchy nor painful.

It develops a few days to a few weeks after a tick bite and is likely to be the first sign of Lyme disease. The rash most often continues to get larger over a period of time and will grow to be well over 2 inches, possibly 8 to 12 inches or more, and may last for several weeks. This rash may sometimes develop a pale appearance in the center, causing a bulls eye shape. Making this even more complicated is the fact that so many with early Lyme disease do not develop the tell tale rash and have to rely on symptoms only.

Either during the time of the rash or shortly thereafter, other symptoms of Lyme disease may appear, which resemble these common flu-like symptoms: fever and chills, malaise (achiness), headache, and achy joints.

The rash and/or the above flu-like symptoms may indicate early Lyme disease and you should see your doctor. When recognized during this early stage, most infections can be adequately treated.

If the above symptoms do not occur, are not recognized, or are not treated properly, then one might develop late Lyme disease, which can more severely affect different parts of the body, such as the joints, the nervous system, and the heart, to mention a few. At this stage, months if not years of antibiotic treatment may be necessary.

It is also reported that greater than 50 percent of those with chronic Lyme disease have co-infections with other Lyme-like organisms, such as Babesia, which contribute to a more severe illness, more symptoms, and a longer recovery.

The bottom line is that whether you are aware of a recent tick bite or not, if you develop an unusual, unexplainable rash or if you develop flu-like symptoms (without respiratory symptoms), especially outside of the flu season, you should visit your doctor and discuss the possibility of Lyme disease, as well as other related diseases.

# Meningitis

Recently, a well known local high school coach made the news with the announcement that he had been admitted to a hospital for treatment of viral meningitis. Thankfully, other than feeling very miserable for awhile, he has had a full recovery.

So just what is meningitis? It is an inflammation of the *meninges*, which is the membrane that surrounds the brain and spinal cord. It is usually caused by an infection from a virus or from bacteria. Although not very contagious, meningitis can be spread by very close contact with someone who has meningitis. It is spread via respiratory droplets from sneezing, or coughing or, in young children, the germs can be passed through the stool.

Viral meningitis is more common and is the least serious. It rarely has any complications. It is treated by taking care of the symptoms either at home or, if necessary, in the hospital.

Bacterial meningitis, on the other hand, can only be treated in the hospital with an intravenous antibiotic. If not treated, or if treated too late, this bacterial infection can lead to brain damage or, rarely, death.

Meningitis is most often caused by germs from a cold or sinus infection, but can also be caused by germs that have entered the blood stream from other areas of the body. As with most contagious diseases, the best ways to lessen the chance of spreading infection are to wash hands frequently, cover your cough or sneeze, and try to stay healthy through proper exercise, diet, and rest.

Most cases of viral meningitis occur in the young. In the past bacterial meningitis also affected the young, but the last few decades, as a result of protection caused by routine childhood vaccinations, the average age at which bacterial meningitis is diagnosed changed from 16 months to 25 years.

The most common symptoms of meningitis are:

- High fever

- Stiff neck

- Severe headache

- Nausea and vomiting

- Lethargy/confusion

- In infants: poor feeding, constant crying, and excessive sleepiness or irritability

The most important test for diagnosing meningitis is the spinal tap. This procedure brings up some dreaded images for most people. In the hands of a competent experienced health care provider, a spinal tap is relatively painless. Other than a possible temporary headache, there are usually only rare complications from a spinal tap. This is the only way to confirm the diagnosis of meningitis and to help guide the treatment of this disease.

Of special note is a type of bacterial meningitis caused by the germ called meningococcus. This also spreads from an upper respiratory infection entering the bloodstream. This is very contagious and mostly affects those living in crowded conditions, such as college students living in dormitories, as well as at boarding schools, and military bases. Pediatricians recommend that all children between the ages of 11-18 should receive the meningococcal vaccine and booster to prevent this serious infection.

# Pertussis (Whooping Cough)

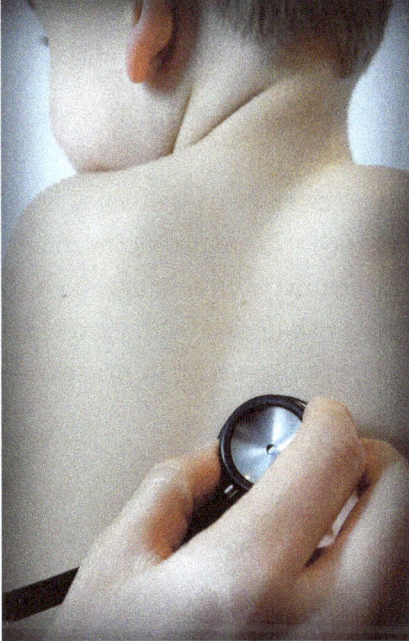

Pertussis, also called whooping cough, is a highly contagious infection of the lower respiratory tract involving the lungs. It usually manifests as a mild persistent cough but can advance to a severe cough. Often in children this cough is followed by a high-pitched breath that sounds like "whoop," thus the name whooping cough.

Pertussis is caused by a germ which is a bacteria and not a virus. It is passed from an infected person who sneezes or coughs, therefore spreading infected tiny droplets into the lungs of anyone who may be nearby. Once in the lungs, the germs can cause an infection, thereby creating inflammation and narrowing of the lung's breathing tubes. This produces the cough and the characteristic whooping sound.

Infants are particularly vulnerable because they are not fully immune to whooping cough until they've received at least 3 immunization shots. This leaves those 6 months and younger at greatest risk for catching the infection. The pertussis vaccine one receives as a child wears off in 5 to 10 years, leaving most teenagers and adults susceptible to the infection during an outbreak. Also, more parents are choosing not to vaccinate their children, thus lowering the number of immunized individuals. This, coupled with the fact that newer vaccines are less potent than the older ones, has increased transmission of pertussis.

The diagnosis of pertussis is often delayed or missed in infants because early symptoms are often mild and the serious cough may not begin for days or even weeks later. A severe infection in infants can be fatal, although thankfully this is rare.

One must consider pertussis for anyone with a cough lasting more than 2 weeks, especially when the person generally feels well, coughs worse at night, and has prolonged coughing spells.

The vaccine for pertussis is combined with the tetanus and diphtheria vaccines, which are routinely given to children in their first years of life, and to adults every 10 years.

Besides infants, those who especially need the vaccine protection are pregnant women in their 3rd trimester because they will soon have contact with their unprotected infant. Mothers have been found to be the greatest source of transmitting whooping cough to the newborn. Infants can also be protected by vaccinating those people who have close contact with them. This "family" protection has been highly successful in protecting susceptible infants.

Tests are available to diagnose pertussis. The decision whether or not to test should be left to your doctor

Antibiotics can be effective especially when given soon after symptoms begin. After several weeks of symptoms they are much less effective. Family members can also be prescribed preventative antibiotics. Pertussis is caused by bacteria and can usually be treated with an antibiotic, but if you just have a bad cough from something like routine bronchitis, which is caused by a virus, antibiotics are not effective. Your doctor will be able to determine the proper diagnosis and treatment.

Bottom line: I recommend to immunize your children and keep immunizations up to date for yourselves.

# Pneumonia

Pneumonia is a potentially serious infection of the lungs.

As opposed to bronchitis, which is a relatively non serious infection of the lungs' airways, pneumonia infects the tissue of the lungs, filling the tiny air sacs with pus and other liquid. This reduces the amount of oxygen reaching the bloodstream.

Germs have the potential of spreading from the infected lung tissue into the rest of the body, causing septic shock and possibly death. Although this is not the common outcome, it still accounts for 60,000 Americans dying of pneumonia every year.

Pneumonia symptoms can vary significantly, depending on underlying health problems and the type of organism causing the infection.

More than half of pneumonias are caused by a variety of viruses. These are usually not serious and often last a relatively short time. Because a person with viral pneumonia tends not to be as sick as someone with bacterial pneumonia, such a person is usually "up and about," and therefore is often referred to as having "walking pneumonia."

Symptoms of viral pneumonia include cough, fever, muscle pain, and fatigue. Signs which often occur with bacterial pneumonia include shaking chills, high fever, chest pain, and cough. Mucus may be present with either type of pneumonia but is more likely with the bacterial variety.

Pneumonia can be contagious. It can occur fairly suddenly in an otherwise healthy person, or it can proceed from bronchitis.

One of the most common symptoms I see in patients with any form of pneumonia is the extreme fatigue, which can last many weeks after all other symptoms have cleared.

Risk factors for pneumonia are as follows:

- Age – Adults 65 and older and very young children
- Chronic disease, such as emphysema, diabetes, and heart disease

- Smoking
- Recent hospitalization, surgery, or traumatic injury

Pneumonia treatments vary on the type and severity of the illness. Bacterial pneumonia will be treated with antibiotics. The entire course of antibiotics must be taken to prevent relapse and to prevent resistant strains of bacteria. Viral pneumonia technically doesn't need antibiotics, but because of the difficulty of distinguishing between the two, a health care provider will usually choose to err on the side of treatment, especially because viral pneumonia can sometimes turn into a bacterial infection.

In all cases of pneumonia, one also needs to control fever, drink lots of liquids, and get plenty of rest.

Prevention of pneumonia is possible. Because pneumonia is a common complication of influenza, getting a flu shot every year is a good idea.

There is a false assumption held by many that getting a pneumonia shot will prevent one from getting any type of pneumonia. Although pneumonia vaccines are available, they are only effective for the common pneumococcal pneumonia germ.

To reduce the risk of pneumococcal pneumonia, two vaccines are recommended for people age 65 and older: Prevnar 13 first, followed by Pneumovax a year later. It is also recommended to vaccinate babies and children younger than 2, and people aged 2-64 who have high risk conditions such as a compromised immune system. Recommended vaccines for children include Prevnar 13 in a series of booster shots in the first two years of life. These recommendations may change over a period of time, so I suggest you seek guidance from your doctor.

It's a good idea to seek medical care if a person has a cough with shortness of breath, chest pain, chills, fever, or feels much worse after a bout of cold or flu. Pneumonia is a serious infection, but for the average person, if it's caught in time and treated properly, it should cause no lasting harm.

# Rabies

Rabies is an infection caused by a virus. It is usually passed on to humans through the bite of a rabid (rabies infected) animal. Rarely, it can be transmitted if the saliva of an infected animal comes in contact with a break in the skin, such as a scratch, or with mucus membranes, such as our eyes, mouth, and nose.

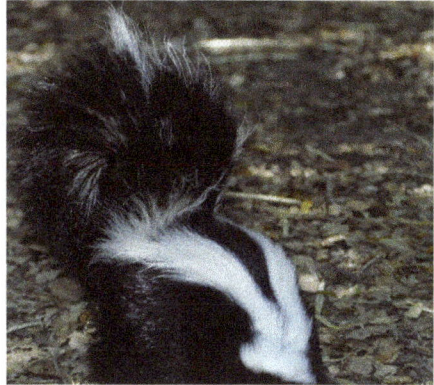

Once the virus enters a body, it travels along a nerve to the spinal cord and brain where it causes encephalitis (brain infection). Once this happens it is usually 100% fatal. That's what makes this such a serious, although thankfully, rare disease. Although it may take one to three months for symptoms of rabies to show up, immediate treatment is necessary.

Rabies causes up to 35,000 deaths worldwide each year, mostly in developing countries. Due to effective animal control and vaccination programs begun in the 1940s, the incidence of rabies in our domestic animals in the U.S. has decreased dramatically. Dogs and cats now account for only 3% of animal rabies. Contrary to common thinking, cats are more rabies prone than dogs. However, the incidence of rabies among wild animals has increased and poses our greatest concern.

To show how rare this disease is, the last case of human rabies reported from an exposure in California occurred in 2003. Although any mammal can be infected with rabies, in California it is usually found in bats, skunks, and to a lesser extent, foxes. It is extremely rare in rodents, such as squirrels, rats, mice,and chipmunks.

How to tell if an animal has rabies:
- A wild animal that seems unusually tame or unafraid and approaches you
- Nocturnal animals such as bats and skunks that are found outdoors during the daytime

- Pets which develop difficulty eating, drinking, walking, or acting unusually strange

- Bats that are unable to fly or have been caught by a domestic dog or cat

If you have been bitten by a possibly rabid animal, wash the wound immediately with soap and water. Your only option for immediate treatment is going to a local emergency room. These facilities stock a medication called "human rabies immune globulin," which is an injection, which must be given as soon as possible after a rabies exposure. This will protect your body from developing the infection. At the same time you will be given the first of four necessary rabies vaccines over the course the next two weeks. These shots are given in the arm. This is a vast improvement from the much feared older method of giving 20 to 30 shots in the abdomen.

After the initial emergency room treatment, I would advise that you immediately call your health insurance provider to see if the next four vaccine shots will be covered by insurance, and if so you could go to most any urgent care clinic for the necessary treatment. For those without insurance, many local county health clinics also stock the necessary post exposure vaccine.

Remember that the timing of proper treatment is critical. Act as soon as possible.

# Shingles

Shingles is a painful rash caused by the *varicella-zoster virus*, which is the same virus that causes chicken pox. Anyone who has had chicken pox may develop shingles. After an episode of chicken pox, the virus can remain inactive, often for decades, in cells of the nervous system. Shingles is caused by a reactivation of the virus, which can manifest as a painful rash always on only one side of the body. The rash can be found on almost any part of the body, but is usually a band of blisters from the middle of the back to the middle of the chest. Pain often occurs several days before the rash. Less commonly one can have just the pain and not the rash.

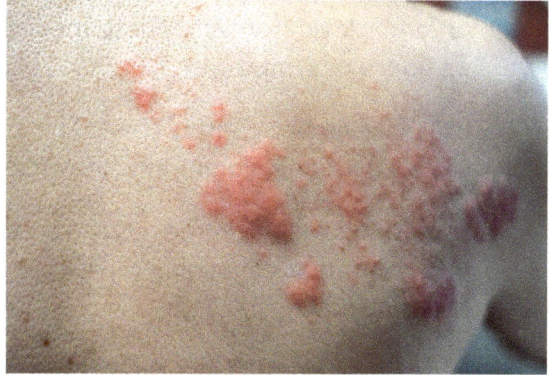

Most of the time shingles occurs only once, but if it does happen again it's usually on another part of the body. About 20 percent of people will develop shingles during their lifetime. Shingles can affect people of all ages, but is more common in those over 50, and much less common in younger individuals. It is sometimes more common in those who have conditions that weaken the immune system, such as medical treatments involving the use of cortisone, chemotherapy, and radiation. Shingles is not life-threatening. A full recovery of shingles is usually expected within a month or two, although one may rarely have a complication called post herpetic neuralgia. This condition causes the skin to remain painful and sensitive to touch for months, or even years after the rash disappears.

Shingles cannot be passed from one person to another, but a person with shingles can pass the virus to a susceptible person causing chicken pox. This usually occurs through direct skin to skin contact with the blisters of a shingles rash.

There are several treatments available from your health care provider:

1.  High doses of an anti viral drug to reduce the duration and intensity of the symptoms. Such medications include acyclovir (Zovirax), valacvclovir (Valtrex) or famciclovir (Famvir). These medicines work best when given within the first 72 hours of symptoms.

2.  Pain relievers to control pain. This usually involves some form of a narcotic such as hydrocodone, commonly known as Vicoden or Norco.

3.  Sometimes helpful in more severe cases of shingles is the application to the rash of an ointment containing capsaicin or a skin patch containing the numbing drug lidocaine.

4.  Because shingles affects the nervous system, it may require a prescription of Neurontin for those experiencing severe pain.

5.  Home treatment of the shingles rash involves keeping the rash clean with soap and water, applying cold wet compresses to the blisters, and for those not taking prescription pain medicine, Tylenol or Advil may be helpful.

There are preventions available in the form of vaccines. All children should be routinely vaccinated for chicken pox as should any adult who has never had chicken pox. Although this vaccine doesn't guarantee to prevent either chicken pox or shingles, it can reduce the intensity of the disease and lessen the chance of complications. There is also available a vaccine specifically for shingles, called Zostavax. It is indicated for those 60 years and older. In studies of people who were given the vaccine, the incidence of shingles infection was reduced, and in those patients who did develop shingles, the severity and duration of infection was lessened.

The bottom line is that if you have a painful rash, it is better to seek treatment from your health care provider sooner rather than later.

# Sinusitis

Sinuses are air pockets found in the bones of the skull. There are seven sinuses which are located on both sides of the nose, between the eyes, and one deep behind the nose. Their true function is not well understood, but it is thought by some that sinuses serve to lighten the weight of the skull, humidify the air we breathe, and to create resonance to our voices.

Acute sinusitis is an inflammation of the sinuses. This in turn causes the lining of the sinuses to become swollen. This swelling interferes with drainage of sinus fluid, thus filling up the sinus, which causes the typical pain. It is usually triggered by the common cold virus and less often by seasonal allergies (hay fever).

Sinus infections affect more than 30 million adults in the U.S. every year and cost the health care system about $3 billion to diagnose and treat.

Risk factors for sinusitis include:
- Hay fever or any allergic condition that affects the sinuses
- Exposure to pollutants, such as cigarette smoke
- A nasal passage abnormality, such as a deviated septum or nasal polyps

Common symptoms of a sinus infection are:
- Nasal obstruction with drainage of thick yellow or green mucus
- Pain, tenderness, swelling, and pressure around the eyes and/or aching in the upper teeth
- Reduced sense of smell and taste
- Cough, often worse at night

Reasons to see your doctor immediately for a sinus infection are:

- Fever greater than 100.5°F (38°C).

- Unbearable facial pain

- Swelling and redness around the eyes and nose

Recommendations for treatment to relieve the symptoms include:

- Saline nasal irrigation— over the past few years since I have become familiar with this treatment, I have seen countless patients with sinus infections that may have needed antibiotics, cure their infections with saline irrigation. "Neil Med" sells a rinsing system that can be found at all pharmacies.

- Decongestants— Over the counter medication such as Sudafed (have the pharmacy tech help you find the one with the ingredient "pseudoephridine"). Nasal sprays such as Neo-Synephrine or Afrin, neither of which should be used for more than one week. (Remember to always read the labels on medications before using them)

# Tetanus

Tetanus is a disease caused by a toxin [poison] produced by the germ *Clostridium tetani*, which produces stiffness and spasms of skeletal muscle. It often begins in the muscles of the jaw, hence the name "lockjaw." Years ago people could die from tetanus due to the jaw locking, leaving them unable to eat or breathe. Fortunately in this age of modern medicine, tetanus infections can be successfully cured.

The tetanus germ is actually quite fragile. It cannot live in the presence of oxygen and does not survive well outside of the human body. It does, however, produce spores [seeds] which are extremely resistant to adverse conditions. These spores are widely distributed in soil and in the intestines of many domestic and farm animals. The spores can also be found on skin surfaces, as well as on many inanimate objects in our environment. The tetanus germ itself is not harmful, but it produces one of the most potent toxins known. This toxin is what causes the severe muscle spasms. Tetanus is not contagious from person to person and antibiotics are ineffective, as they have no effect on the harmful toxin.

The tetanus germ enters the body through any type of open wound. The incubation period ranges from 3 to 21 days, usually about 8 days. The deeper the wound, the less oxygen is present and the tetanus spores proliferate spreading the toxin throughout the bloodstream. Tetanus may follow puncture wounds, especially stepping on a nail. A rusty nail is only slightly more dangerous than a non rusty nail only because its surface is rougher and more likely to harbor germs. Burns, bites, and even minor scratches can also lead to tetanus. Occasionally the victim may not even recall a preceding injury.

Tetanus immunization came of age during World War II. Tetanus fatalities fell from thousands per year to just a few cases a year. Almost all reported cases of tetanus are in those who have never been vaccinated, or those who were properly vaccinated but have not had a booster in the preceding 10 years.

Routine tetanus immunization begins after birth at age 2 months and is a series of 4 doses with a booster at about 5 years of age prior to entering school. From then on a booster is needed every 10 years throughout one's lifetime to maintain adequate protection. Receiving a booster sooner than necessary is not harmful. Better safe than sorry. Tetanus vaccination is almost 100% effective and unlike the old horse serum used years ago, the new variety being used rarely causes any serious adverse reactions. The most common problem for some after receiving the tetanus shot is a sore arm, with occasional redness and swelling around the injection site. This will resolve on its own and is not an allergic reaction.

If you have sustained an open wound to the skin:

1.  Clean the wound with soap and water and receive a tetanus vaccination as soon as possible if:

    •  You've never had one before

    •  If the wound is very dirty and deep and your last booster was more than 5 years ago.

    •  If the wound is relatively clean and minor and your last booster was more than 10 years ago

2.  Have your health care provider keep you up to date with a booster every 10 years.

# Upper Respiratory Infection (Common Cold)

Everyone has at one time or another experienced a common cold manifested by such symptoms as nasal and sinus congestion, runny nose, mild sore throat, and cough. This common infection may last from a few days to one to two weeks. It is always caused by a virus and therefore patience, and not antibiotics, is the main treatment.

Bronchitis can be thought of as any cough that is not caused by pneumonia or asthma. The main symptom of bronchitis is a cough without a fever. People with bronchitis usually just have a cough and do not feel particularly sick and are able to continue their normal daily activities. One can expect coughing from bronchitis to last from one to three weeks. Again, this is almost always a virus infection and antibiotics are usually not necessary. If a cough does last more than several weeks, or is associated with fever, it would be wise to visit your doctor.

Sinusitis is an infection of the sinuses, which are air-filled pockets around the nose in the skull.  This infection is usually preceded by a common cold. It too is usually caused by a virus, but after lingering for one to two weeks may turn into a bacterial infection. One of the key factors in determining the proper treatment for a sinus infection is the duration of the symptoms. If you have had a cold for one to two weeks, and are experiencing pain or pressure in the sinuses along with yellow or green nasal mucus, and perhaps a fever, then antibiotics may be helpful.

A sore throat is often a symptom of a cold, but can sometimes be a bacterial strep throat infection. A good rule of thumb is that if a sore throat is associated with a bad head cold, and especially with a cough, it is usually caused by a virus and needs no prescribed treatment. If, however, one has a sore throat without cold symptoms or cough, but does have a fever and a past history of prior strep infections, then the most likely culprit is the strep germ, which needs to be treated with antibiotics. Strep is much more common in children than in adults.

Over the counter medications for adults can be helpful in alleviating the miserable symptoms of respiratory infections.  The following are the basic ingredients of all the myriad combinations of cold and flu drugs found on pharmacy shelves:

- Acetaminophen (Tylenol) or ibuprofen (Advil) may be used to reduce fever and to alleviate aches and pains

- Pseudoephridine (Sudafed) is a decongestant to help relieve nasal and ear congestion

- Guaifenesin (Robitussin or Mucinex) is an expectorant to help loosen mucus (Dinking lots of liquids may work just as well)

- Dextromethorphan is a cough suppressant which may help ease a persistent cough

One may purchase a sinus rinsing system called Neil Med, which can be found at all pharmacies. This is a natural treatment using a salt based solution to mildly flush out the sinuses helping to clear out the mucus as well as acting as a decongestant. I have found this to be one of the very best treatments for bad colds and sinus infections.

See your doctor if you have a fever for more than 3-4 days or if your fever is 103°F (39.4°C) or higher. Your doctor will determine whether antibiotics are necessary to treat you. At the very least, your doctor may prescribe medication that will help to alleviate your symptoms and make you feel more comfortable.

## Influenza

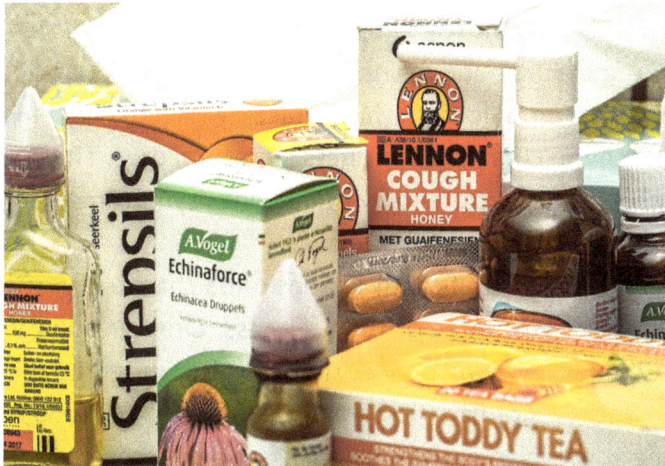

Influenza, often called the flu, is a virus affecting the respiratory tract, causing illnesses ranging from symptoms of a severe cold, to life threatening infections such as pneumonia. It often affects up to 10% of the entire population and is associated with an average of 36,000 deaths a year throughout the United States. Most deaths occur in the very elderly, the very young, or in those with chronic illnesses.

Influenza is transmitted by direct and indirect contact via respiratory droplets from coughing, sneezing, or from just shaking hands. The incubation period is several days and contagiousness can last as long as a week after the symptoms begin. The best way to limit its spread is by frequent hand washing with soap and water for 15 to 20 seconds, and by limiting close face to face contact with others when symptoms are present. It is very important to know the difference between the common winter cold and influenza.

As opposed to a common cold, influenza has these distinguishing characteristics:
- Very sudden onset
- Fever
- Aches
- Sore throat

At the onset of influenza symptoms people often say they feel as if they had been "run over by a truck."

The treatment for influenza is mostly symptomatic care:  plenty of rest, Tylenol or Advil (ibuprofen) for fever and aches, and maintaining adequate liquid intake. There are drugs such as Tamiflu, available from a doctor, which if taken within the first 48 hours of influenza symptoms may shorten the course of the illness by several days. These are recommended for the elderly or chronically ill patients with influenza symptoms.

Being immunized by a flu shot significantly lessens one's chance of getting the flu. As with any treatment, there is no guarantee of 100% success. One can still get a bad viral upper respiratory infection during the winter months even after receiving the flu vaccine. Most people who receive the flu shot have no bad reaction to it. Some people may experience redness and swelling at the injection site lasting a few days. One cannot get the flu from a flu shot because it is made from a deactivated dead virus. The benefit of the flu shot far outweighs the minimal risks. Although the ideal time for a flu shot is from mid-October through November, the flu season can extend through May.

# Influenza Questions/Answers

I'd like to answer common questions I hear about influenza and the flu shot.

1.  *I'm afraid I'll catch the flu from the shot.* You cannot catch the flu from the flu vaccine. These vaccines are made with viruses that are killed (inactivated), and cannot cause an influenza infection.

2.  *I've had the flu shot previously and I got the flu anyhow.* This is possible in that no vaccine is 100% effective.

3.  *I've never had a flu shot and have never had the flu.* Consider yourself lucky, and as in most cases, one's luck will usually wear out. Don't take a chance, this could be the year.

4.  *The flu is no big deal.* Tell that to those who have not survived a bout of influenza, or to the worker who misses a week or more of work, as well as the student missing time from school. Besides, having the flu can make you feel very miserable.

5.  *I worry that it could be harmful to my baby/child to have yet another vaccination.* Babies have a higher incidence of death due to influenza. There is no proof that the flu vaccine worsens or changes the effects of the other routine childhood vaccinations. The recommendation is that everyone from 6 months of age and older should receive the flu vaccine.

6.  *I have already have a chronic disease and I take lots of medications. Do I really need a flu shot too?* All the more reason to receive a flu shot since flu is the most deadly for those with chronic medical conditions.

7.  *I have a tremendous fear of getting a shot.* Easy to say but this is probably the time to work on the principle of mind over matter.

8.  *I'm pregnant, won't a flu shot harm my baby?* Not only has the flu vaccine injection been proven to be safe during pregnancy, but is highly recommended for pregnant women in any trimester of pregnancy.

9.  *I'm 35 years old and healthy, do I really need a flu shot?*  In 2009-2010, the swine flu (HINI virus) took a particularly heavy toll on the age group 18 to 64 years of age. Better safe than sorry.

10. *Any reason I absolutely shouldn't get a flu shot?*  There are a few reasons, the most common being a prior allergic reaction to a flu shot. The vaccine should be delayed if you have an illness with a fever.

11. *When should I get the shot?* The flu season typically begins as early as October and can last until late spring. It takes about 2 weeks after receiving the shot for it to become effective.

12. *Where can I get a flu shot?*  Most major pharmacies provide flu shots on a drop-in basis, as well as through most primary care doctor's offices. Larger medical groups have special drop in flu clinic days. For children, call your child's primary care provider to find out how they are to receive a flu vaccination.

13. *How much will a flu shot cost me?*  For most people it is free either because they have a government insurance plan such as Medicare or Medicaid, or they have private insurance. For those who have no such coverage, the out of pocket cost of flu vaccine is between $30-$50.

## Animal Bites

Animal bite statistics to consider:

- Over 3,000,000 animal bites occur each year.

- Over 300,000 animal bite related visits to emergency rooms occur each year, costing approximately $160 million dollars.

- 80% of bites are from dogs, 10% from cats and remaining 10% from other animals.

- Children are the most frequent victims of dog bites, especially 5-9 year old boys.

- At least 50% of dog bites come from family or neighbor's dogs.

- Men are more frequently bitten by dogs than women (3:1) and women are more frequently bitten by cats (3:1).

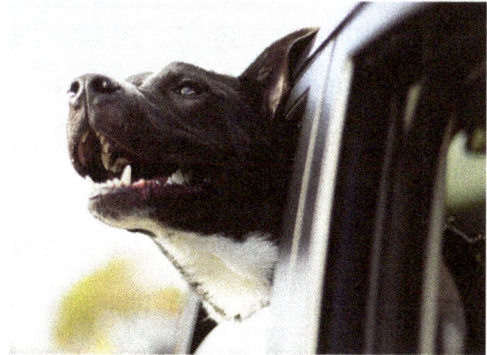

The law in most municipalities, requires that the local animal control office be contacted when any person or animal is bitten by another animal, whether the biting animal is wild or domestic.

In many states, when a bite victim seeks medical treatment, the treating physician must also, by law, fill out an animal bite form and send it immediately to animal control. This is true even if the bite is from one's own pet. An animal control officer will investigate the incident and advise the animal owner about a quarantine of the animal, which, is usually done at the owner's home.

In general, dog bites cause less infection than cat bites. This is because dog teeth are more dull and less able to penetrate a victim very deeply, while cat teeth are shaper, proportionally longer, and able to penetrate deeper. Infections are often evident in less than 24 hours. Bites to the face, although cosmetically worrisome, are least prone to infection and bites to the hands/fingers are most likely to become infected.

Seek medical treatment immediately for a bite anywhere on the body by any biting animal if:
- Wound is gaping, (wide open)
- Wound won't stop bleeding (Always apply pressure first)
- You have cosmetic concerns
- You have a weakened immune system
- Wound already appears infected
- You need a tetanus booster

I want to emphasize that if you have suffered what you believe to be more than just a superficial bite to the hand from any source, dog, human, or especially cat, see your doctor for wound evaluation and treatment as soon as possible. You will most likely be treated with antibiotics before an infection develops. Hand infections, especially from bites, if not treated promptly and aggressively may be a cause for hospitalization.

# Bicycle Accident

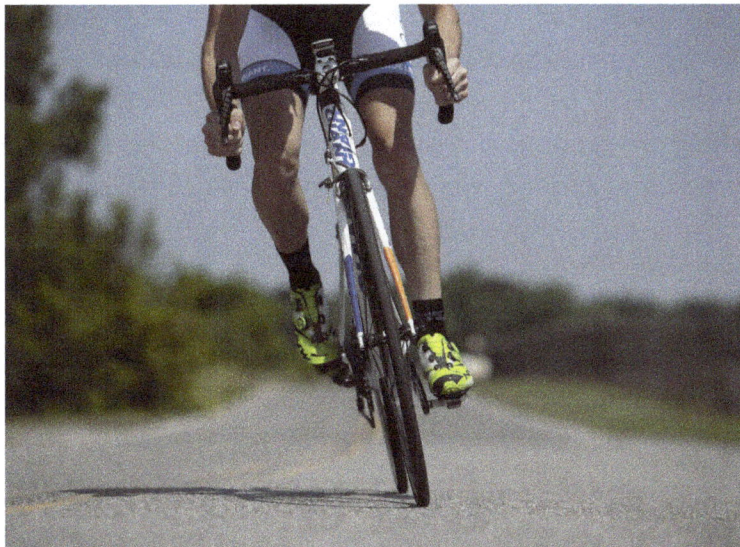

I was out for my routine bike ride. The pavement was unusually wet due to a light rain during the night. As I got close to the top of my ride, I suddenly realized that I had mis-judged my timing and had to get back home, so I quickly turned around and headed back in just a little more of a hurry. I came to a sharp curve in the road and as I made the turn I saw a car in the opposite lane. Although there may have been no problem with this, my reaction was to hit the brakes, which locked up on the wet pavement, and down I went. I ended up on my back partially on top of my bicycle. And yes, I was wearing my helmet.

I was able to pedal back home feeling just a little achy and decided not to tell my wife about what had just happened, since I don't think she's ever gotten over my ladder accident several years ago when, once again, I almost killed myself. When I arrived home and got off my bike I realized that my right hip was hurting and I was limping a little. I couldn't hide that from my wife, so I fessed up. She actually took it in stride. However, within a few hours, my hip hurt so much that I couldn't walk on it.

An X-ray of my hip thankfully showed no evidence of a fracture, but it took several weeks on crutches to recover.

The reason I'm telling this story is to remind my fellow weekend warriors and risk takers that accidents happen in a split second and are usually caused by a momentary act of carelessness such as my ladder and bike accidents. Even at my age, I'm beginning to learn to be a little more cautious and careful with my activities. Coincidentally, both of my accidents occurred in unusually wet environments, which should have made me even more careful.

I find that, for myself and the thousands of patients whom I have treated over the years for a wide variety of injuries, doing any activity in even just a little more of a hurry than usual or trying to take even a little short cut, or not being fully aware of our surroundings, are the common denominators for causing injuries. Almost every patient I treat for an injury, including myself, uses the word "stupid" when describing how their injury occurred.

Do yourselves a favor and exercise just a little more caution and patience in all your activities. Take it from someone who's learning it the hard way.

# Head Injuries (Concussion)

There has been much attention recently given to the potentially serious injury to the brain from suffering a concussion. For school kids who are at significant risk of learning disabilities, emotional or behavioral changes, and memory problems, the focus of recovery should be mental as well as physical rest.

From babies to high school students, children with concussions make nearly 144,000 visits to emergency rooms each year, and a significant number of these injuries go unrecognized and are not reported.

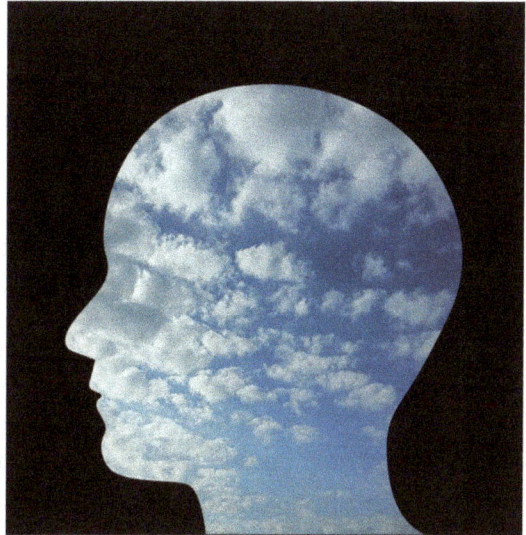

Younger athletes may be at a greater risk of damage from a concussion because their brains are not fully developed. When athletes take a hit to the head in football, are slammed by an elbow in soccer, or fall from a bike or skateboard, their brains get banged against the inner walls of their skulls, thus causing the injury commonly referred to as a concussion.

Common symptoms of a concussion are:

- Loss of consciousness, no matter how brief

- Headache

- Vomiting

- Memory loss or behavioral changes especially confusion or feeling "foggy"

Children with the above symptoms or any other worrisome symptoms that parents or adult guardians are concerned about after a head injury, should prompt an immediate medical evaluation at a facility best suited for this, such as an urgent care clinic or hospital emergency room. The evaluating physician may order a CAT scan of the head depending on how serious the signs and symptoms are.

It can no longer be acceptable for a head injured athlete, young or old, to "shake it off" and get back into the game. Our young athletes must be instructed to immediately report any head injury. Coaches and trainers have become more aware of the potential dangers, both short and long term, of traumatic brain injuries, and are having the injured players seek immediate medical evaluation.

Especially dangerous is the "second impact syndrome" when a player receives a second significant head injury within a short time of the first injury. This can lead to even more serious health consequences.

Those of us in the medical profession, who are dealing with head injuries, are using protocols to help return the athletes to their routine activities. The focus of recovery is rest, both physical and mental. The injured athlete needs to be eased back into all routine activities. A medical reevaluation should be performed before allowing a return to contact sports.

The bottom line is that head injuries in athletes need to be taken very seriously because of both immediate and potential long term consequences. Mental rest after the injury is just as important as physical rest. Although this article focuses on sports related head injuries, the principles I have discussed pertain to anyone with a head injury no matter what the age of the individual or the cause of the injury.

# Hot/Cold Therapy

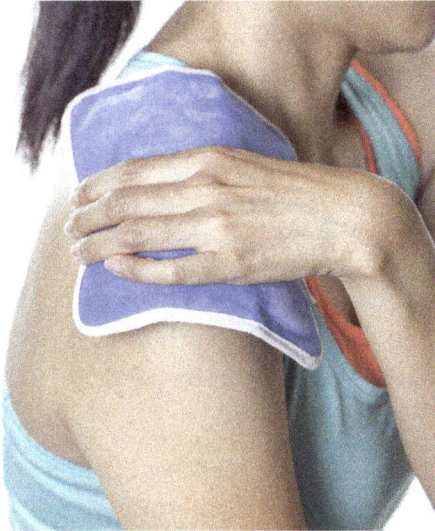

A common question is when to apply either hot or cold packs to treat injuries and pain.

Acute injuries are usually accompanied by pain, swelling, and tenderness, whereas chronic injuries often manifest as lingering pain from an acute injury, or from overuse of muscles and ligaments from too much exercise or heavy work. Our necks, backs, shoulders, and knees are common sources of ongoing pain. Chronic pain may come and go, whereas acute pain from a recent injury is usually constant.

The use of ice is somewhat controversial in that although the cold slows down the blood supply to the injured area thus possibly reducing swelling, it also inhibits the healing properties in the blood being brought to the injured area. I think ice is good for pain and swelling of an injury if it is used immediately for no more than 15-20 minutes at a time every hour or two for the first day only. Using ice longer or more frequently is probably not necessary. Icing can be done by applying ice in a plastic bag, gel packs (from a pharmacy), or even from using a bag of frozen vegetables.

Heat treatment may begin within a day after the injury. It works by opening up blood vessels and helps by increasing blood flow to the injured tissue, thus easing the pain. The word heat is defined as very warm to comfortably hot, but not too hot. Heat can be applied by using a hot water bottle, a heating pad, a gel pack, or a hot soak in the tub. Be very careful using heat if you have diabetes or poor circulation as you may cause burns to the skin.

The use of products to apply to the skin overlying a painful body part, such as "Deep Heat" or "Mentholatum," work by causing the skin to feel cool and then warm. These feelings on the skin distract you from feeling the aches and pains deeper in the tissue. This may be helpful for minor aches and pains.

Both hot and cold compresses should be wrapped in a thin towel so that you neither burn nor freeze the skin. Be aware that you may burn your skin if you fall asleep on a heating pad. Hot or cold packs should be used for 15-20 minutes at a time. For ice treatments I recommend repeating every 1/2 to one hour, if convenient, and for heat, every 2 to 4 hours.

In summary:

- Use a cold pack as soon as possible for  immediate injuries such as sprains of the ankle, wrist, knee, back, or any other injured joint or body part. Cold treatment should usually be stopped within 24 hours.

- Use a hot pack for a painful injury after the first day, for recurrent pain from previous injuries, or as a warm up of painful areas prior to exercising.

# Ladder Injuries

It finally caught up with me. After 40 plus years of climbing ladders (mostly to get on my roof), I recently fell off of one and injured myself. In the middle of a nice relaxing Sunday afternoon, I decided to climb my extension ladder and get up on my roof to reposition a plastic tarp. Now, you must understand that over the past 37 years, I have treated hundreds of patients (mostly men) for injuries from falling off a ladder. Therefore, I have always promoted ladder safety and felt that I have been very cautious when getting up and down on a ladder.

On this particular occasion, I climbed the ladder on my back deck to my one-story flat roof. I did what I set out to accomplish and started back down the ladder. I cautiously placed my first foot on the top rung of the ladder. I then started to bring my other foot to the rung and suddenly I knew something bad was about to happen. I was going down. In a split second, and with absolutely no chance of saving myself, I ended up falling.

The ladder base had slipped away from the house, and I fell straight backward, landing 10 feet below, flat on my back, on top of the ladder. I felt like I had broken my back, it hurt so much. I laid there on top of my ladder for a few minutes; no one else was at home (another critical mistake). I realized that I could move my legs and arms, so at least I knew I wasn't paralyzed. After a while, I managed to get up and hobble into the house. I felt like passing out from the pain and the shock to my body.

My injuries turned out to include a broken right ankle, a cracked rib below my shoulder blade and a severely bruised and swollen lower back. The next day, I ended up with a cast on my leg with instructions to not place any weight on that leg for 4 to 5 weeks. I had to get used to hobbling around on crutches (not a pleasant experience), while dealing with a pretty painful back. Improvement came slowly, but surely.

Over 2 million people suffered ladder injuries from 1990 to 2005. That amounts to about 135,000 injuries a year. (I'm sure there are many more that are not reported.) The majority of ladder injuries happen at home and mostly to men over age 40.

Injuries include but are not limited to:

- Death

- Permanent disability. (From paralysis, pain, or serious head, neck, or back injury)

- Temporary disability usually from a broken arm or a leg

- Painful arthritis in later years as a result of these injuries

- Loss of income

- Loss of recreational activities

- Loss of intimacy

My ladder safety recommendations:

- When you think about climbing a ladder, consider whether doing so is worth the risk of possible serious injury or disability

- NEVER climb a ladder when no one else is at home

- ALWAYS have another responsible person to work with you, to secure the base of the ladder and to be your conscience when you're attempting to do something stupid (come on guys we all do it) while up on the ladder

- Check out ladder safety websites online for information on proper ladder placement and safety

To you ladder climbers out there, please read and think long and hard about what I have written. Women, show this article to your men. If it can happen to me, it can happen to anyone. Don't kid yourself. I thank God I'm alive after my accident. I see how easily, in a split second, I could have died or become permanently disabled. That just wouldn't have been fair to my wife, my children, or to anyone who cares about me.

Ladders are not casual tools. They are as dangerous as a loaded gun, so use them with appropriate caution and respect.

# Youth Sports Injuries

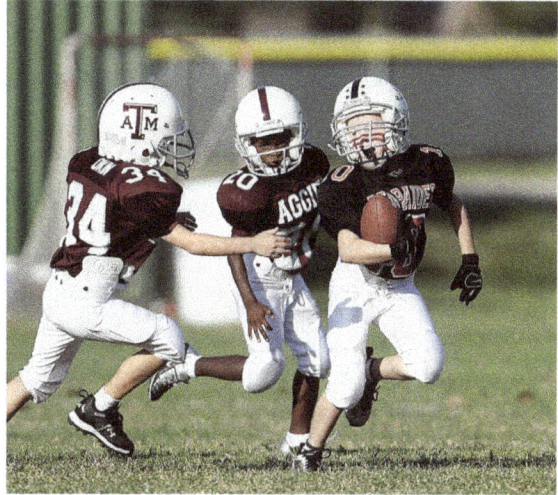

As a new school year begins, your child may be one of the estimated 50 million children participating in organized sports throughout the country. Sports programs are great in teaching the children about teamwork, competition, and providing much needed exercise. However, statistics show that 1 in 3 of these children will be injured enough to miss a practice or a game, and over a million are expected to visit an emergency room this year for a sports related injury, with medical expenses costing over a billion dollars a year.

The majority of organized sports related injuries occur during practice rather than games. The top sports for injuries are football, basketball, soccer, baseball, volleyball, wrestling, cheerleading, gym, and track and field.

The most common injuries are to the head, face, fingers, knees, and ankles. The most common injury diagnoses are sprains/strains, fractures, contusions/abrasions, concussions, lacerations, and dislocations.

Concussions in particular, have received much attention recently and appropriately so. There is no longer any doubt about the short term and potential long term dangers of this injury, especially to the young developing brain. We now have very specific guidelines about when to allow a child with a head injury to return to games or practices, as well as how best to treat a child with a significant head injury/concussion.

Symptoms of a concussion are loss of consciousness no matter how brief, headache, vomiting, memory loss, and behavioral changes, especially confusion and/or feeling "foggy."

Any of these symptoms necessitate prompt medical attention.

There are also the overuse injuries involving tendons, bones, and joints. This is due to playing the same sport and performing the same movements too often, too hard, and at too young an age without adequate rest and recovery.

Sports related injuries are inevitable, but there are some things that can be done to help prevent and treat injuries. Be sure your child is involved in a sports program that is properly maintained and adequately coached. Coaches should be certified in CPR and have a plan to respond to emergencies.

Make sure your child has and uses proper gear for a particular sport in order to reduce the chance of injury.

Encourage your child to perform warm up and cool down routines prior to and after sports participation. The warm up will make the body's tissues warmer and more flexible, and the cool down will loosen muscles that may have tightened during exercise.

Be sure your child has access to adequate liquids during exercise and while playing. Emphasize the importance of maintaining hydration to prevent dehydration and heat illness.

Encourage liberal use of sun screen to protect the skin from the sun's damaging rays and help to prevent future melanoma.

Get professional help if you think your child's injury is serious, such as when you suspect a fracture or dislocation of a joint, severe pain, or swelling.

Statistics show that only 1 in 4 young athletes become elite players in high school and only 1 in 1600 high school athletes go on to professional status. Therefore, the emphasis in youth sports should be in the enjoyment and long term involvement in exercise and sports. Remember to match your child's abilities to the sport, and not to push him or her too hard into a sport they may not like or be incapable of doing.

## Bee Stings

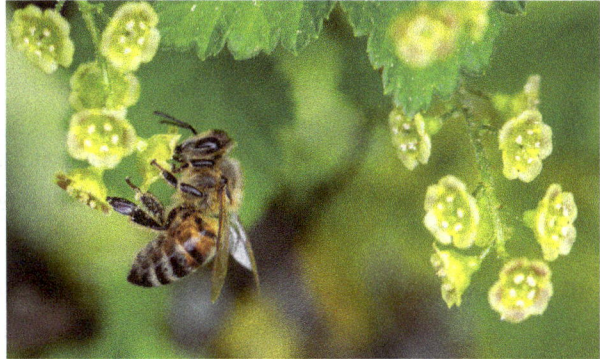

Our most common local stinging insects are yellow jackets and bees. Yellow jackets are attracted to our delicious picnic food and are more aggressive than bees. They sting defensively when they feel that their nests are threatened. They also sting when stepped on, sat upon, or have in some way been provoked. If one is being attacked by many bees or yellow jackets, it is best to vacate the area and run away as fast as possible. These insects are capable of flying up to 15 miles per hour and pursuing for distances of 50 to 100 yards. So don't run too slow or stop too soon!

Wasps, including yellow jackets, can sting multiple times and leave no stingers in its victim. The honey bee sacrifices its life with its sting because it leaves the stinger and part of its abdomen with the venom sack attached to the skin of the victim. This stinging apparatus continues injecting venom into its victim for up to one minute after the sting. This is why the new accepted method to remove the stinger is just to pull it out with your finger tips as fast as possible. Trying to take the time to find something to scrape off the stinger as was previously recommended just wastes time, and allows more venom to be injected at the sting site. Tests have proven that pinching out a stinger doesn't force out more venom.

Stings are exceptionally painful. The best local treatment is to immediately place an ice pack on the sting site for up to several hours. Home remedies such as applying pastes of meat tenderizer, clay, toothpaste, aspirin, and baking soda, have no proven benefit. Taking an antihistamine, such as Benadryl by mouth, may help with itching.

A local toxic reaction to the venom occurring within hours to days after the sting may involve redness and swelling of just a small area around the sting, or a much larger reaction often involving an entire arm or leg. As bad as this may seem, it is not serious or life-threatening, and will resolve on its own in a matter of days. These reactions are sometimes mistaken for a secondary infection, but this is very rarely the case and anti-biotics are hardly ever necessary. A sting on the face may cause worrisome swelling, but is not dangerous. However, a sting inside the mouth or throat can be quite serious and needs prompt emergency treatment.

Almost every person who is stung will have at least a mild reaction around the sting site. Less than one percent of the population will have a severe allergic reaction.

Serious allergic reactions may occur within minutes or up to several hours after the sting. Usually the more serious the reaction, the sooner the symptoms begin. For those who have suffered a serious reaction to a sting, I would recommend a consultation with your doctor who may recommend allergy shots to make one less sensitive. An inject-able adrenaline kit such as an "Epipen" may be prescribed to those who have had a very serious prior sting.

What to do when stung:

1.  Pull stinger out as fast as possible by any method; using fingers is now allowable

2.  Remove self from vicinity of stinging insects as fast and far as possible

3.  Apply ice compresses to sting

4.  Take Benadryl by mouth as soon as possible

Call 911 if you experience:

- swollen tongue or throat
- difficulty swallowing
- tight breathing
- feeling faint
- severe hives

# Head Lice

With the return of students to school, we are facing the issue of head lice. These creatures have adapted themselves quite well to all societies throughout the world. Children are most commonly affected from interaction with other students as well as the use of shared combs, headphones, and beds. This condition, officially called *Pediculosis capitis,* is second only to the common cold as the most common communicable illness in school children. Lice are not dangerous and do not spread disease. Socioeconomic level is not a great factor in the occurrence of this condition. Girls are affected more commonly than boys, but hair length has not been reported as a factor.

The head louse is an insect 3-4 mm in length. Its lifespan is about one month. The female deposits eggs in a sack, which is then cemented firmly to the base of a hair follicle. These attached eggs called *nits*, will hatch in 8 days. They rapidly mature and soon begin feeding on blood through the scalp. They do not jump, fly, or live on our pets.

The main symptom of lice infestation is itching of the scalp. The diagnosis is made by identifying the lice or nits. Nits are more visible than the actual lice. They are tan colored when they contain live eggs. When the nits are empty they are white, resembling dandruff, but are much more difficult to remove. The back of the scalp above the neck is the most likely place to find evidence of head lice.

There are several ways to treat head lice. The most natural method is called wet combing, which is a welcome alternative to using insecticides, and the safest treatment for those under two years of age. Combing is performed with a fine tooth comb. The hair should be wet, with an added lubricant such as a hair conditioner or olive oil. Combing is done until no lice or nits are found. Repeated combing can be done every 3 to 4 days for several weeks.

For children over the age of two, the most effective method for treating head lice is the use of topical insecticides. The most commonly used is Permethrin cream rinse 1 percent, sold over the counter by the name Nix. This is a relatively safe product when used as directed. The scalp should be shampooed, rinsed with water, and towel dried. Then Nix is applied and allowed to remain in the hair for 10 minutes before being washed out with water. A second treatment may be given in 7-10 days if live lice (not nits alone) remain. Hair should still be combed as described above to remove the nits. If the lice problem persists, see your doctor and discuss treatments available by prescription.

Washing contaminated clothing and bedding is important. Lice can survive free from the scalp for up to two days, so vacuuming carpets and furniture is helpful.

The most common causes of treatment failure are not following through with the treatment and continued contact with others who are infested. Household members should be inspected and treated if necessary. Our local schools have a "No Nits" policy, meaning that students remain out of school until all nits are gone from the scalp. This again demonstrates the importance of combing nits out of the hair.

There is no need to panic over head lice. This condition can be cured with proper treatment and patience. If all your efforts seem in vain, see your doctor for further help.

# Spider Bites and Stings

The subject of "bites and stings" has always been of interest to me in my practice over the years. In particular, I have tried to educate patients about the brown recluse spider. Many have come to me with an open sore on their skin, attributing such a lesion to a brown recluse bite. Others also know stories of friends or family who have had horrendous brown recluse bites. Doctors have diagnosed and treated patients for brown recluse bites on the assumption that the bite was caused by the brown recluse. This spider bite does have the potential to cause a large open sore, sometimes leading to treatment with a skin graft.

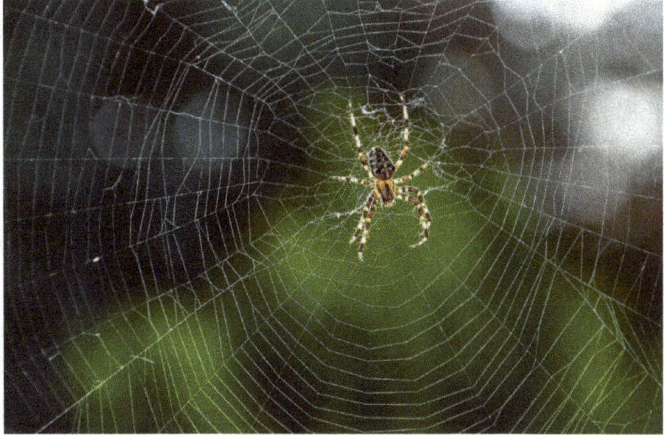

The fact is that the brown recluse spider does not live in California. It is native mostly to the central southern states and to the lower Midwestern states. Less than 10 specimens have ever been positively identified as brown recluse in California and there is usually some connection between the spider and a recent move or shipment of goods from the southern states.

Every story about the brown recluse I have ever heard is anecdotal and not based on the positive identification of the spider. In the areas where the spider is in its natural habitat, it is usually found in groups and not as isolated specimens. They are very shy and "reclusive" and as with almost all biting spiders, they will only bite when threatened. The most likely source of a bite in its natural habitat is from someone putting on clothing in which the spider has been hiding.

So what causes a skin wound that is mistaken for a brown recluse bite? Bites from other spiders and insects, as well as localized infections of the skin from other causes, would top a long list of conditions causing such similar appearing lesions.

What spiders do we need to be concerned about? The bad news is that almost all spiders are technically poisonous. The good news is that of the tens of thousands of species of spiders, only about twenty of them are capable of biting a human. Most have mouth parts too small or weak to penetrate human skin. It is reassuring that virtually all spiders are essentially non aggressive and do not deliberately bite humans. The likelihood of a spider lurking in our bedding or dropping onto us from the ceiling is very remote.

The black widow spider is very common in most locales. I would venture to say that every house has a black widow spider hiding under or behind something in the garage, attic, basement, storage shed, etc. These spiders are also non-aggressive and usually have to be provoked to bite a human. Black widow bites are very rarely fatal and probably cause death less often than from a lightning strike. The most common symptom of a black widow bite is muscle cramps, especially involving the abdomen, which can mimic appendicitis.

Many people live in an area with scorpions that sting and tarantulas that bite. Neither one of these in most locales is lethal; however, an encounter with either one can be very painful. It is also a fact that daddy-longlegs spiders are non-poisonous.

In general, we humans have a great fear and disgust of spiders. We squash them, sweep them out, and smother them with pesticides. Spiders are actually beneficial to humans in that they eat many insects especially those that are carriers of disease or are disgusting to us such as cockroaches, mosquitoes, and earwigs. I think that little Miss Muffet should have held her ground and not been "frightened away."

## Generic Drugs

"Billions wasted on pricey drugs" was the headline in the newspaper this week. Medicare claims that the program is wasting hundreds of millions of dollars because doctors continue to prescribe, and patients continue to ask for pricey name brand drugs when cheaper generic drugs are available.

What exactly are generic drugs? They are copies of brand name drugs which have the same dosage, side effects, intended use, risks, strength, and safety of the brand name drug. In other words, the brand name drug and the generic version of it should be identical.

The generic version of a drug can be manufactured and sold once the patent on the brand name drug has expired. The generic costs much less than the brand name drug mainly because the generic manufacturers don't have to duplicate the hundreds of millions of dollars spent on research, development, and marketing conducted by the original manufacturer.

There is concern by many that generic drugs are cheaper because of a compromise in quality or effectiveness. However, the Food and Drug Administration requires that the generics be as safe and effective as the brand name drug. The generic must be bioequivalent to the name brand product, which means that the amount of active ingredient is delivered to the body at the same time, and used in the body in the same way as the brand name. The generic will often be a different color, shape, or flavor than the brand name and it also may have different inactive ingredients, but the active ingredients must always be the same.

There are a few classes of drugs, such as anti-seizure medications, thyroid hormone replacement, and blood thinning drugs, when it is best not to switch back and forth between generic and brand name versions. Your doctor can explain this in more detail.

Patients do, for the most part, have a choice of generic versus name brand drugs, but must realize that both private and public insurance plans may not pay for the non-generic, or will require a higher co pay, thus increasing the out of pocket cost of the drug. Feel free to discuss this with your doctor and pharmacist.

# Medical Marijuana

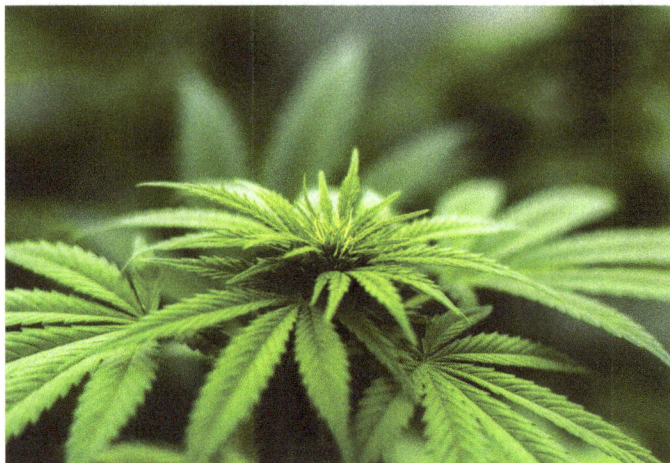

Marijuana has been used for medicinal purposes for several thousand years beginning with the ancient Chinese. It was used at that time for a multitude of medical problems, from the treatment of malaria to the treatment of constipation.

Marijuana was introduced to the United States in the mid 1800s and was prescribed by physicians for its therapeutic benefits until 1937, when it was prohibited from being prescribed. Then in 1970, it became legally prohibited for anyone to even possess or use marijuana.

Because of public demand for the medical use of marijuana in California, in 1996 it became legal to use for medical purposes and soon other states followed suit.

The benefits of marijuana are attributed to its cannabinoid compounds, of which over 100 have been identified. The 2 most researched and well known of these are tetrahydrocannabinol (THC), which has some medicinal qualities but is also the main component for the mind altering effects of marijuana, and cannabidiol (CBD), which causes much less of a high and is used for its medicinal purposes

Most patients smoke the dried plant for the quickest results. Marijuana's active ingredients can also be delivered through capsules, vaporizers, liquid extracts, foods, and beverages. One major problem is that dosing can be unpredictable since the level of active ingredients varies between plants, as well as the fact that absorption of ingested forms varies among patients.

Although many users have found multiple benefits from marijuana for the treatment of numerous health problems, there are really only of few that have passed scientific testing. They include:

- Nausea, especially when caused by cancer chemotherapy and AIDS
- Chronic pain especially when due to neuropathy, cancer, or AIDS
- Glaucoma
- Multiple sclerosis
- Epilepsy
- Appetite and weight loss in cancer patients

Again, I want to emphasize that there are a myriad of other conditions that may be helped by marijuana, but are currently not backed up by scientific evidence. Most medical practitioners would prefer that patients first use traditional proven treatments for most health problems and to use marijuana in situations where treatment has failed.

There are known health risks to the use of marijuana including:

- Impairment of thinking, problem solving skills, and memory
- Increased anxiety and panic attacks
- Reduced balance and coordination
- Increased risk of heart attacks, inflammation of heart muscle, and atrial fibrillation
- Possible hallucinations and withdrawal symptoms
- Lowering of blood glucose and blood pressure,  and increased risk of bleeding

Smoking marijuana, which is the most common method of use, has its own set of potential problems. It is associated with possible increased chronic bronchitis and lung cancer (although much less likely than smoking tobacco).

At this time experts recommend limiting the use of medical marijuana to adults older than 18 years of age. There are also other health related conditions when marijuana should not be used including:

- History of schizophrenia or other psychiatric disorders
- Severe heart or lung disease
- Severe liver or kidney disease
- Pregnancy, or planned pregnancy, and when breast feeding

Even with the possible side effects and the non-uniformity of doses and strengths of its various forms, I would encourage the use of medical marijuana for the known conditions where it has been proven to be helpful. I can also accept its use in any number of conditions when more conventional treatments have failed.

As marijuana use becomes more widely legalized it should open the door to much needed research which would provide more information as to the best doses and delivery systems for medical use, as well understanding the risks and benefits for all users. This information would be of great help to both physicians and patients.

# Opioids

There's been much in the news recently about opioid addiction. The use and abuse of opioids has skyrocketed in recent years, and has become a truly nationwide problem. The most common opioids are Vicodin (hydrocodone), OxyContin (oxycodone), Dilaudid (hydromorphone), and Demerol (Meperidine).

Opioids are used to reduce pain, especially when over-the-counter pain medications, such as Tylenol or Advil are ineffective. Opioids are powerful pain killers that block messages of pain to the brain and decrease the brain's perception of painful discomfort. The problem is that they also cause a feeling of euphoria. Opioids are great for short term pain management, such as after an injury or surgery. Opioids are also useful for long term pain, such as from cancer. For long term pain other than cancer, their benefit is debatable, especially since taking opioids for 4 weeks or longer puts one at risk for dependence and addiction.

Side effects of opioid use include nausea, constipation, itching, and drowsiness. Stopping opioids after more than short term use can cause withdrawal symptoms such as nausea, vomiting, depression and diarrhea.

A major concern is that recently some 33,000 Americans fatally overdosed on opioid pain medication. More people die from drug overdoses than from motor vehicle accidents.

The other problem we're experiencing at an alarming rate today is the use of heroin for those who started their addiction on opioids. The reason for this seems to be that heroin is cheaper and more readily available than are opioids.

Don't be alarmed if your doctor prescribes an opioid. More than 95% of patients won't have a problem taking opioids. One concern is teenagers who are prescribed opioids after painful dental procedures especially wisdom tooth extraction. Studies have shown that teens treated with opioids after wisdom tooth extraction have a significantly higher chance of later opioid abuse. Discuss this with your dentist and monitor your child's use of opioids.

Don't try to decrease your addiction risk by cutting down on your dose and waiting until the pain gets so bad that you have to take the medicine. This can actually increase the risk of addiction.

Here are suggestions to keep in mind when taking opioids from your doctor:

- If necessary, have a family member help you to make sure you're taking only the prescribed dose.
- Keep opioids in a lockbox to help prevent them from getting into the wrong hands.
- Keep expectations realistic; total pain relief is rare even with opioids.
- Avoid alcohol or other sedatives while on opioids.
- Safely discard opioids when they are no longer needed or have expired.

Opioids are appropriately recommended mostly for short term and occasionally long term pain relief. Work closely with your doctor to obtain the most effective and safest use of opioids.

# Over-the-Counter Cold and Flu Medications

Almost all of the hundreds of products available over-the-counter contain at least one or a combination of the following ingredients:

1. Tylenol (acetaminophen) or Advil (ibuprofen) for aches and pains

2. Sudafed, a decongestant, containing either pseudoephedrine or phenylephrine

3. Guaifenesin an expectorant (thins mucus)

4. Dextromethorphan, a cough suppressant

5. Antihistamines, such as diphenhydramine or chlorpheniramine

We could probably get by with only five different bottles of cold medications on those pharmacy shelves, each containing one of the above medications. I think that taking these drugs individually rather than in combination is better so that one can tailor one's symptoms to a specific medication and avoid taking something that might not be necessary. Always read the label on the medication package to check on potential interactions with drugs you may already be taking and to know the possible side effects or warnings.

Here's how these drugs work. Tylenol or Advil work equally well for relieving the aches and pains of an illness, as well as helping to reduce a fever. Read the directions carefully. The maximum daily dose for acetaminophen is 3000 mg. per 24 hours. The maximum adult dose for ibuprofen is 800 mg. which can be taken up to 4 times a day.

Sudafed, for those who do not have high blood pressure, may be helpful to relieve the swelling of the nasal/sinus passages and to relieve the pressure in the ears due to blocked eustachian tubes. Sudafed, with the main ingredient pseudoephdrine, has changed from over-the-counter to behind-the-counter, and it will need to be signed out for purchase through the pharmacist. It's probably worth the effort. Sudafed with ingredient phenylephrine can still be purchased over-the-counter, but may be a bit less effective than the pseudoephridine.

Guaifenesin is an expectorant, which means it helps to thin out mucous in the nose and sinuses, as well as in the lungs. Dextromethorphan is a cough suppressant that should help at least a little to lessen one's cough. Honey has also been found to be effective in slowing down a cough. Neither of these remedies is strong enough to actually stop a cough and will not interfere with the healing process.

Antihistamines are really most useful for the symptoms of allergies like hay fever, but they may help colds by slowing down mucous production. Perhaps they help most by their side effect of drowsiness, thereby helping one to sleep.

Another highly effective way to decongest the nose and sinuses is to perform sinus rinsing using either a netti pot, or my preferred method, a Neil Med sinus rinsing kit found at most pharmacies. I have found rinsing to be highly effective to alleviate sinus symptoms and to even treat or prevent sinus infections.

In Summary:

- For aches and pains from a cold or flu, use Tylenol or Advil
- For stuffy nose, sinus congestion, or plugged ears, use Sudafed
- To loosen mucous use guaifenesin, such as Mucinex or Robitussin
- To help slow down a cough, use a medication with dextromethorphan, such as Robitussin DM or Vicks 44, or try a couple tablespoons of honey in a hot beverage
- Get plenty of rest and drink lots of liquids

Closely follow the directions for proper dosage found on the medication labels.

These are some basic guidelines for choosing medications for the symptomatic relief of common cold and simple flu. The effectiveness of these drugs is somewhat limited, but worth trying. Adequate rest, liquids, and time still play a major role in recovery from these miserable conditions.

See your health care provider if you have a fever for more than a few days, if you have a fever of more than 103°F at any time, or if you have any significant concerns about your illness.

# Over-the-Counter Pain Medications

Does your back ache? Do you have a headache, toothache, or sprained ankle? What medication should you choose for pain relief? In most cases these types of pain are common and can be treated with over-the-counter pain medications, which make up a 2 billion dollar a year industry. The few basic medications available to treat your pain must be chosen wisely, and you must be aware of the possible side effects of these drugs so that they don't cause more harm than good.

The potential for harm rises with increasing doses of the medication and in taking it for long periods of time. The elderly and those with chronic medical conditions face a greater chance of experiencing troublesome side effects.

In spite of the pharmacy shelves being filled with a mind boggling combination of available pain relieving drugs, they are really all made up of any one of the following types of drug:

ACETAMINOPHEN (Tylenol)

This is probably the safest of the drugs when taken at the recommended doses. It is classified as an analgesic (pain reliever), as well as a fever reducer. It can be used by all ages, except infants  with fever under 3 months of age who should see their doctor for evaluation and treatment. It can have a toxic effect on the liver and should be used very cautiously, if at all, by those with liver disease or those who drink more than 3 alcoholic beverages a day. A big advantage of acetaminophen over the others is its tendency not to irritate or harm the stomach. It can be taken if one is also taking a blood thinning medication. Follow the dosing directions carefully.

IBUPROFEN (Advil, Motrin IB)

This is called an anti-inflammatory analgesic because it acts not only on most any type of pain but also on inflammation. Many people use this medication for relief of soft tissue aches and pains associated with vigorous exercise or hard physical labor. Like acetaminophen it is very effective as a fever reducer for young and old. Do not use in infants under 6 months of age without consulting your doctor. Unlike acetaminophen, it does not harm the liver in recommended doses, but it can be very irritating to the stomach, possibly leading to bleeding and/or stomach ulcers. Long term high dose usage has been linked to increase risk of heart and kidney disease. It should not be taken while taking a blood thinning drug.

## NAPROXEN SODIUM (Aleve)

This is also an anti-inflammatory drug taken for the same indications as ibuprofen. It can be taken less frequently than ibuprofen and still achieve the same benefit. It causes similar side effects to ibuprofen with perhaps less likelihood of stomach and kidney problems.

## ASPIRIN (Bayer, Excedrin)

This time honored drug is also an anti-inflammatory, analgesic, and fever reducer. Under the care of a physician, it is now being used in a low dose to help prevent heart disease. It's cheap and plentiful, but has more potential side effects compared to the others. It is more frequently associated with stomach irritation and bleeding. It is not recommended in children less than 16 years of age. Because of the potential side effects, I personally would not take aspirin to treat routine pain unless there was no other choice.

The bottom line is that if you have mild pain for whatever reason, any of the above drugs could be helpful. Results vary for each individual. Pay close attention to the various side effects, which I have listed and which can be found on the medication label. Be sure to see your doctor if you get no pain relief from these commonly used medications or if your pain lasts more than a few days.

# Pill Swallowing

On occasion I have patients present to me with the sensation that a pill was stuck in their throat. This is not an uncommon occurrence. A number of people do have problems swallowing medication in tablet or capsule form. When a pill actually does get stuck it is usually not really in the throat, but in the upper esophagus just below the throat.

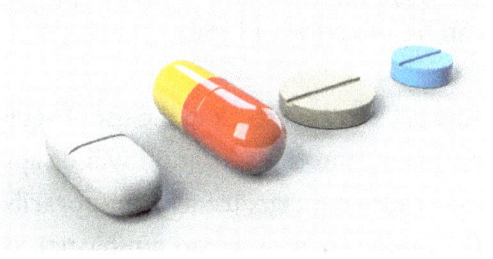

Certain conditions involving the esophagus will predispose one to having difficulty swallowing pills, such as strictures (narrowing), scleroderma (hardening), and a condition called *presbyesophagus* where the muscles of the esophagus do not function properly.

Warning signs of a stuck pill are:

- Feeling of a tablet or capsule stuck in the throat

- Pain with swallowing

- Achy dull pain in chest after swallowing a pill

There are techniques that help one to swallow pills more easily:

- Relaxing and taking several deep breaths before swallowing

- Taking several sips of water prior to swallowing a pill to help lubricate the throat

- Cutting large pills (not capsules) in half after consulting with your pharmacist to be sure it's OK to do this. Use a pill cutter purchased at your pharmacy rather than a kitchen knife.

- Do not lie down shortly after taking your pill or it will be more likely to get stuck in your esophagus. This is especially true when taking medicine just before lying down to sleep at night.

Pills and capsules can also be more easily swallowed when mixed with food. If you have trouble swallowing them whole, pills can be crushed and mixed in most any type of food.

Capsules can be opened and sprinkled on food. They can be mixed with small servings of applesauce, pudding, or flavored Jello. Some pills are time released and should not be crushed. Again, check with your pharmacist to ensure that your particular pill or capsule can be mixed with food.

Any pill that gets stuck in the esophagus will usually dissolve within one to two days causing no harm, and the sensation will disappear. There are a few pills worth mentioning that may cause damage, usually temporarily, to the esophagus. These are aspirin, doxycycline (a commonly prescribed antibiotic), potassium chloride, vitamin C, and iron. On rare occasions one of these stuck pills can cause an ulcer or a more dangerous perforation (hole) in the esophagus.

The same advice, with approval from the pharmacist, can be used for children's medication, which is usually prescribed as a liquid. It can be made more pleasant tasting when mixed with chocolate syrup, ice cream, jelly, or jam without decreasing its effectiveness.

When picking up your prescription medication, before you leave the pharmacy, take a close look at the label on each container. Make sure it has the following:

- Your name, as well as the prescribing doctor's name

- The name and phone number of the pharmacy

- The date it was prescribed

- The name and the amount of the medication

- Simple understandable directions

- The expiration date

- The number of refills, if any

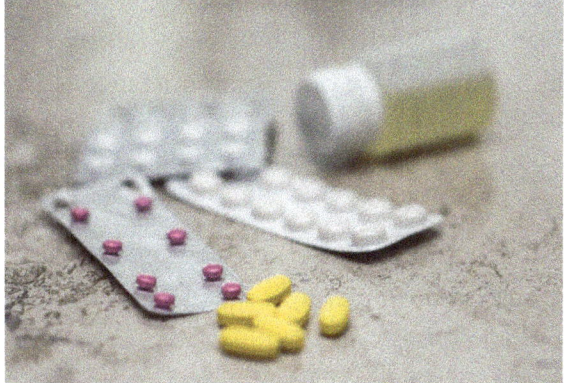

When you arrive home with your medication, be sure to keep it in its original container in order to prevent any future confusion. An exception to this rule would be to put the medication in a weekly pill container, which is the best method of helping to remember to take medication on schedule. These containers can be purchased at your local pharmacy. You may dispose of the cotton plug, which is often found in the container. Always keep containers tightly closed. When bringing a new medication into your home, take time to dispose of any medication, which has expired or has been discontinued by your physician.

Take time to read the drug information given to you by the pharmacist. This is usually a fairly detailed computer print out of information you need to know before taking your first dose. Spending time to read this information will help you to understand how often and when to take the medication, what side effects may occur, whether to take the drug on a full or empty stomach, and whether it needs to be refrigerated.

It's probably safe to say that most people who have prescription medication are not aware of proper storage techniques. Heat and humidity are the greatest factors in the deterioration of stored medications, especially tablets and capsules. The medicine cabinet in the bathrooms is actually the worst place to store medication because of the high heat and humidity. A cool, dark, and dry location, such as a top dresser drawer or a high shelf in a closet is preferred. Keeping them out of the reach of children is of utmost importance. Also of equal importance is to keep controlled drugs, especially narcotics, in a locked secure location. Do not store medication in the glove box of your car as the intense summer heat will cause rapid deterioration.

What actually happens to medication which is beyond the expiration date? In almost all cases the drug merely loses its potency, but does not become dangerous or toxic. One notable exception to this rule is common aspirin, which when it breaks down forms acetic acid (vinegar) and salicylic acid, which are stomach irritants. Regardless of the expiration date, if at any time you open a medication container and it either looks or smells different from how you remember it, either dispose of it properly or have your pharmacist check it out for you.

Discard any medication which has:
- Expired
- Been discontinued by your doctor
- No label on the container
- Changed color, smell, or seems different from how you remember it

Medications which should be safely discarded include prescription drugs, over-the-counter medications, pet medicines, vitamins, medicated creams and ointments, and liquid medication in containers.

In many states it is now illegal to discard medicines and sharps by flushing them down the toilet or throwing them into the trash. Most local pharmacies will accept unwanted medications and sharps, which should be transported in an approved safe container that can be inexpensively obtained from the participating pharmacy.

# Prescription Medication Part 2

Many people are taking more than one medication, seeing more than one doctor, or have more than one health problem making it essential that you and your doctor are aware of all the medications you take, as well as understanding any possible drug interactions that may occur. When seeing your doctor, bring all your medications or a list of medications you are currently taking.

It is very important to read the information given by the pharmacist when picking up your medication. This information can describe possible drug interactions. These interactions, which often cause unwanted side effects can occur as:

- Drug to drug interactions: when two or more drugs interact with each other such as a sleeping pill (a sedative) taken with an allergy medication (an antihistamine)

- Drug to food/beverage interactions: food can interfere with drug absorption

- Drug to health condition interactions: taking the decongestant Sudafed when one has high blood pressure can significantly raise the blood pressure

- Drug to over the counter medication interactions: taking an antacid and drug together can block the drug from being absorbed from the stomach

One common drug with drug interaction is taking an antibiotic and the effect it has on birth control pills. Medical literature says that antibiotics pose a very small risk of a woman getting pregnant. A woman being advised of this small risk may decide to temporarily use a back up birth control method.

Some medications are altered by what you eat and when you eat. Food may delay or decrease the absorption of the drug causing it to be less effective. Some medications work best on an empty stomach, which means taking it either one hour before eating or 2 hours after eating. On the other hand, some drugs work better when taken with food just after a meal. Your medication label will tell you how to take the medication. If there is no mention of taking it with or with out food, then it can be taken either way.

Patients often ask if alcohol can be consumed while taking medication. The general rule of thumb is that medication and alcohol taken close together may change the potency of a drug making it either less or more potent. The most potentially serious reaction is the combination of alcohol and narcotic pain medications, sleeping pills, and sedatives. Many "accidental" or "suicidal" deaths we hear about in the media are the result of these drugs being combined with alcohol. I do not advise consuming alcohol while taking medication, but I realize that it is a fact of life. If drinking is done in moderation, then it is best that the consumption of alcoholic beverages and the taking of medications be separated by at least two hours.

In summary, when taking prescription medication carefully read the instruction sheet given by the pharmacist, as well as the label on the container. This will help to ensure safe and effective use of your medication.

# Steroids

When hearing the word "steroid" many people think of athletes taking performance enhancing hormone-like drugs. But in the everyday world of medicine, we're talking about a nearly miraculous class of drugs called corticosteroids, which include cortisone, hydrocortisone, and prednisone. These are hormones, which are produced naturally in our bodies by the adrenal glands, which sit on top of our kidneys.

These corticosteroids are mainly helpful in reducing various types of inflammation found within our bodies caused by such diseases as arthritis, asthma, allergies, and many others. They also suppress the immune system, which helps to control conditions in which the immune system attacks its own tissues, such as lupus and rheumatoid arthritis. Corticosteroids also help in the treatment certain cancers and help in preventing rejection of organ transplantation.

Corticosteroids can be administered by mouth via pills or syrups, or by inhaler and nasal spray to treat allergies or asthma. They can also be given by injection to treat local problems, such as tendonitis and local arthritis, as well as given topically as a cream, ointment, or lotion to treat skin conditions, such as poison oak, eczema, and psoriasis.

As miraculous as corticosteroids are, they do have the potential for serious side effects. When taken by mouth they can cause high blood pressure, elevated pressure in the eyes (glaucoma), fluid retention, and weight gain, especially of face, abdomen, and back of neck. When taken longer they can trigger or worsen diabetes, thin the bones and skin, increase risk of infections, and cause bruising and poor wound healing. Inhaled corticosteroids can cause fungal infections of the mouth and hoarseness.

Injected corticosteroids can cause many of the previously described symptoms and should be given no more than 3-4 times a year at your doctor's discretion.

The following are recommendations for the best use of corticosteroids with the least risk. Take as low a dose as possible and for as short a time or perhaps take it every other day. Use a non oral form if possible, such as an inhaler for asthma or a topical form for a skin condition.

If you've been taking corticosteroids for a long time be very careful when stopping. Do not stop abruptly. It must be tapered down to allow the adrenal glands time to recover. Eat a healthy diet and get plenty of exercise in order to maintain a healthy weight and to strengthen bones and muscles.

Working closely with your doctor can take advantage of the wonderful healing effects of corticosteroids while dealing with the known risks.

# Tylenol

I will use the term Tylenol (the most recognized brand name) and acetaminophen (the chemical name) interchangeably in this article. A Federal Drug Administration panel has recently made several recommendations concerning Tylenol and Tylenol containing products. These are only recommendations and are not written in law as of this time. The FDA recommendations are as follows:

- That prescription Vicoden (hydrocodone and acetaminophen) and Percocet (oxycodone and acetaminophen) be very carefully controlled

- That over-the-counter products that contain acetaminophen (there are, at this time, over 600 of such medications) carry stronger warning labels

- Reduce the maximum over-the-counter strength of a Tylenol pill from 500 mg. to 325 mg

What's at issue here is the fact that acetaminophen in high doses can cause liver damage and in very high doses can cause liver failure and death. This problem usually occurs when patients take more than the recommended daily dose of Tylenol or when they take Tylenol plus another combination drug that also contains Tylenol, such as Theraflu or Nyquil, thus unknowingly exceeding the recommended dose.

Since it is well known that alcohol also has a negative effect on the liver, the combination of alcohol and Tylenol consumption together has an even greater negative effect on the liver.

Tylenol has been around for decades and has been consumed by millions of people world-wide for the relief of pain and fever. I believe that when taken in recommended doses it is safe and effective. The alternatives to Tylenol such as aspirin or anti inflammatory drugs such as ibuprofen have their own risks especially in terms of stomach bleeding. The decision to take either Tylenol or an aspirin product is a matter of risk versus benefit. You may wish to speak with your doctor about this.

I agree with the panel's findings and recommend the following:

- Tylenol or its various products should not be used if one consumes more than two alcoholic drinks per day

- The maximum single adult dose should be no greater than 650 mgs. (two 325 mg. tablets)

- The maximum daily dose should be less than the currently recommended dose of 4,000 mg. I propose taking no more than 2800 mg. per day, which is equal to taking two 350 mg. tablets every six hours.

- Always carefully read the label on the bottle of any over the counter medication to see if acetaminophen is one of the ingredients

Be careful but not fearful of Tylenol. For treating pain or fever it is a very useful medication when used properly. Consult your doctor if you have any questions.

## Cell Phones

I recently read an article that talked about a new study that had linked cell phone use and cancer. After some research, I have found many study results that do not support this information. Several large, well-done studies in the United States have found no direct link between cell phone use and brain cancer even in children. However, several of these studies did indicate that further investigation of this possible link is needed.

The sheer number of people using cell phones, estimated at some 350 million users in the U.S. and up to 5 billion worldwide, has prompted concern about its use and human health. Interestingly, brain cancer incidence and mortality have changed little over the last decade and has been linked more to aging than to radiofrequency waves from cell phones.

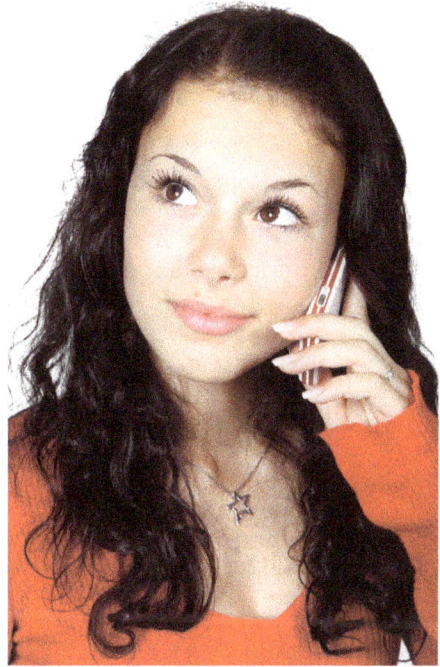

Cell phones emit what is called radiofrequency energy, which is a form of electromagnetic radiation. Unlike X-rays, which because of their high energy have been proven to cause cancer, the energy from cell phones and other similar devices is low energy and actually does nothing more than to generate heat with things with which it comes into contact, which is how microwave ovens work. So, although a cell phone can technically heat up an area of tissue around whatever side of the head the phone is used, it is a minimal change, cannot be detected, and has not been found to be harmful.

Other conditions reportedly linked to cell phone use because of prolonged contact of the phone against the body are saliva gland tumors, acoustic neuroma (a tumor of the nerve that connects the ear to the brain), and male infertility. Sleeping difficulty is another potential problem if the phone is used prior to going to bed.

Other devices that we are exposed to emit similar energy waves as the cell phone. These include Wi-Fi routers, wireless computers, iPads, laptops, etc., and could have similar effects on the human body as the cell phone.

Given all this information, it appears that at this time, in my opinion, there is no conclusive research evidence connecting cell phone use and cancer. But, until more and larger well conducted studies are done, I would still be somewhat cautious. The following are some recommendations found in current literature:

- In general, try to keep wireless devices away from your body as much as is practical, especially keeping the cell phone away from the head by using the speaker phone, ear plugs, or headset

- Text instead of talk as much as possible

- Do not place a turned on device in a pocket or jacket close to your body

- Do not sleep with devices in bed or near pillow. This includes computers and laptops.

- Placing the phone in airplane mode will stop the energy waves

In conclusion, I don't want to be an alarmist, because as I have indicated, at this time there's not enough evidence to link cell phone use and cancer. But I also don't want to look back years from now and wish that we had heeded the above recommendations.

# Human Body Statistics

Hearing about people living to be 100 years old or older made me realize just how amazing the human body is to keep functioning for so many years. I am awestruck by this body of ours that began with just two microscopic cells coming together and developing into a complex living organism made up of some 75 trillion cells. Many of these cells have specialized to perform amazing functions, making us the incredible beings that we are.

I'd like to share with you some interesting statistics about the human body. Let's take an 84 year old person for example. This person:

- Has a heart beating 100,000 beats daily, 35 million beats a year and over 3 billion beats in a lifetime

- Has a heart that has pumped over 48 million gallons of blood in a lifetime, which is enough to fill over 2,000 average sized in ground swimming pools

- Has lungs that breathe 23,000 times daily producing 2,600 gallons of air or almost 80 million gallons per year, which is enough in a lifetime to fill about 160 full sized hot air balloons

- Has two kidneys that produce 1½ quarts of urine a day or over 10,000 gallons per lifetime. These same kidneys have processed one quart of blood per minute, 423 gallons per day, and 13 million gallons per lifetime.

- Has consumed and processed 3½ pounds of food a day equating to over 53 tons of food in a lifetime

- Has produced almost 10,000 gallons of saliva in a lifetime

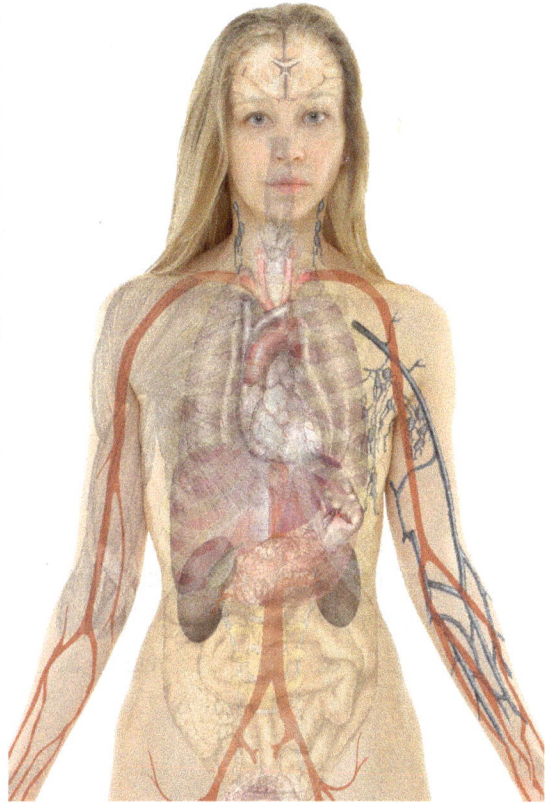

Other interesting facts about our bodies:

- Our bodies are composed of 50 to 100 trillion cells, 300 million cells die and are replaced every minute. 15 million blood cells die every second.

- We have over 650 muscles. The largest is the gluteus maximus (buttock) and the smallest is the stapedius in the middle ear.

- We have 206 bones. The largest at 18 inches is the femur (thigh bone) and the smallest at 1/10 of an inch is the stapes in our middle ear.

- We have about 20 square feet of skin, with 35,000 dead skin cells coming off the body daily, which means our entire skin is replaced once a month. We shed 40 pounds of skin during our lifetime.

- We have 60,000 miles of blood vessels, which would stretch around the world over 2 times

- Our noses can detect 50,000 scents

- We blink 6 million times a year

There are roughly 20,000 diseases that affect the human body and there are over 600,000 physicians representing 150 medical specialties to deal with human health and disease. Take good care of that amazing body of yours.

# Medical Terminology

The following medical terms frequently come up in my conversations with patients. After each medical term is the common word or explanation.

- conjunctivitis / pinkeye
- otitis media / ear infection (in the middle ear behind the eardrum)
- external otitis / "swimmers ear" infection of the ear canal
- pharyngitis / sore throat
- fracture / broken bone
- sprain / stretched ligament
- strain / pulled muscle
- contusion / blunt impact injury often causing a bruise
- hematoma / localized collection of blood
- hemorrhage / uncontrolled bleeding
- laceration / a cut to the skin
- abrasion / scraped skin
- skin abscess / boil
- hordeolum / sty
- cystitis / bladder infection
- pyleonephritis / kidney infection
- cellulitis / a bacterial skin infection
- analgesic / pain relieving medicine
- hypertension / high blood pressure
- arrhythmia / irregular heartbeat
- CPR / cardiopulmonary resuscitation
- myocardial infarction / heart attack

- angina / lack of oxygen to heart causing chest pain
- cerebral vascular accident (CVA) / stroke
- transient ischemic attack (TIA) / mini-stroke
- hemetemesis / vomiting blood
- hemoptysis / coughing up blood
- melena / black blood in stool
- hypoglycemia /  low blood sugar
- cardiovascular / pertaining to heart and blood vessels
- renal / pertaining to the kidney
- hepatic / pertaining to the liver
- cerebral / pertaining to the brain
- cutaneous / pertaining to the skin
- jaundice / yellowing of the skin
- edema / swelling

# Non-Physician Providers

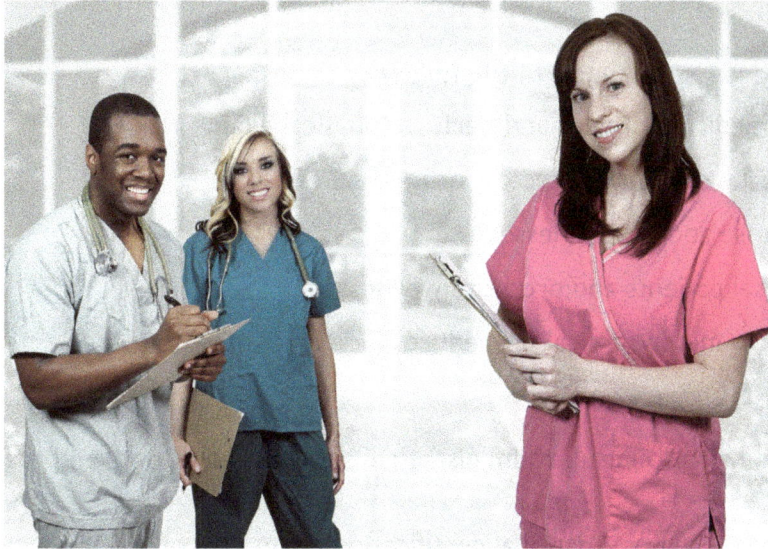

Physician assistants (PAs) and nurse practitioners (NPs) are professionals licensed to practice medicine under the supervision of a physician. They can perform a wide range of medical duties from basic routine medical care to highly technical procedures. They may also work as surgical assistants to a surgeon. Their patients can range from newborns to the very elderly. They can be found in virtually every medical and surgical specialty.

In rural areas, which are short of physicians, they often work independently conferring with a supervising physician as necessary and as required by law. Their responsibilities are determined by their experience, their working relationship with the supervising physician, and state laws.

The first physician assistant program began in 1965 at Duke University Medical Center in North Carolina. Many of the first students in this program were Navy Corpsmen who had received considerable training and on the job experience in the Vietnam War but had no options to use their talents upon return home to the U.S.

The Nurse Practitioner program began at the University of Colorado also in 1965. Nurse Practitioners first receive their R.N. degree and go through further training to practice medicine under a physician's supervision in some states and individually in others.

Both N.P.s and P.A.s can perform the following duties:
- Take medical histories and perform physical exams
- Prescribe medication and order medical tests
- Diagnose and treat illnesses
- Counsel patients and promote wellness
- Perform minor surgical procedures independently
- Assist in surgery

Their practice may also include administrative services, education, and research.

Both groups have to pass a national certification exam, be continually reexamined after a number of years, and also have to complete a prescribed number of continuing medical education hours in order to maintain their licenses.

P.A.s and N.P.s can be found serving a wide variety of medical needs and in various settings from remote rural areas to major urban centers, in physician's offices, hospitals, clinics, armed forces, and government agencies.

I have worked with physician assistants and nurse practitioners for the major part of my career covering some 40 years. They have been a tremendous asset to my practice, as well as to the many physicians who have utilized their talents.

# Urgent Care vs. Emergency Care

Having begun my career in a busy county trauma emergency room (ER) and then having worked in urgent care, I wanted to use this experience as an opportunity to explain how you can decide when to go to the ER and not to urgent care.

Emergency rooms see more than 300,000 patients daily in the U.S. To help diminish this large number of patients, many of whom do not have serious problems, urgent care centers began seeing patients in the late 1970's. There are now more than 9,000 urgent centers functioning across the country and the number is growing.

Because of lower overhead, urgent care centers charge much less for non-emergency care than do emergency rooms where overhead to provide needed comprehensive care is much more expensive.

In general, ERs can use all that the hospital has to offer which includes the ability to admit a patient, especially to the Intensive Care Unit (ICU) for more serious problems. Also, a hospital-based ER is able to utilize state-of-the-art X-ray and imaging studies, as well as a full laboratory, which in most cases can obtain immediate test results. ERs usually have a full complement of specialists on call to take care of a variety of medical, surgical, or pediatric problems.

In general, almost any condition that can be described as "severe" should be treated at an emergency room. Coming to urgent care, even though it may be closer to you than the ER, with such a severe problem often leads to being sent by paramedics to the emergency room. This is not only very expensive but can waste valuable time to begin much-needed treatment. Once you arrive at urgent care, it is the on-duty doctor who determines whether your particular problem can be treated there, or if you need to be sent for more comprehensive care at the ER.

The following are some of the more common reasons to go to an ER rather than urgent care:

If you have severe:

- Chest pain
- Abdominal pain
- Headache
- Backache
- Persistent vomiting and/or diarrhea
- Difficulty breathing and/or shortness of breath
- Burns
- Trauma

Or go to the ER if you have:

- An allergic reaction with trouble breathing, are feeling faint, or have severe hives
- Fainting, sudden dizziness, or weakness
- Sudden changes in vision.
- Confusion, change of mental state, or difficulty speaking
- Suicidal thoughts
- Uncontrollable bleeding (Remember to always apply pressure to the wound until you receive treatment)
- An injury to an arm or leg that causes a deformity, that is to say  an arm or leg that is bent instead of being straight
- Poisoning or drug overdose
- Loss of consciousness
- Miscarriage or a sick newborn baby
- Illegal drug related  problems

Call 911 if you consider an injury or illness to be very serious or potentially life threatening.

# When to Call in Sick

There are certain times of year when respiratory illnesses such as colds, coughs and the flu begin to make more of us ill. I'm frequently asked by patients whether or not they can return to work, school or to resume exercising when feeling sick. I'd like to offer some guidelines to help make such decisions.

I know that missing work or school can put one behind in their workload, but going to work or school while ill can not only prolong one's illness, it can also spread it to others. It seems that employers and educators are becoming more tolerant to excused absences due to illness. They realize that not only will workers/students who are sick not be as productive, but that they may cause others to become ill and affect the entire office or classroom. It has been reported that more than two-thirds of all health related productivity losses are due not from sick people missing work but from sick employees who show up and perform poorly.

I would like to offer some reasons to stay home when ill:
- If you have a fever of 100°F (37.7°C) or higher
- If you have frequent coughing or sneezing
- If you are taking medication that may make you dizzy, light-headed, or unable to concentrate
- If you have vomiting or diarrhea

Consider returning to work or school when the above symptoms have cleared up.

Things one can do whether at home, work, or school to help from spreading illness to others are:
- Wash hands frequently with soap and water or with a hand sanitizer
- Cover your face when sneezing or coughing, using tissue paper or the sleeve of your arm

- Try to stay several feet from face to face contact with those around you
- Keep your hands away from your face

I can't emphasize enough the importance of keeping a distance between those who are sick and others who are not. Germs are spread through respiratory droplets from our noses and mouths. In normal conversation and breathing, those droplets from the mouth may extend out 1- 2 feet from you, but a sneeze or cough can spread them an estimated 6-8 feet. Those who are healthy need to act defensively when in the presence of someone who is showing symptoms of an illness.

Mild to moderate physical activity is usually OK if you have a common cold and no fever. Don't exercise if you have a fever, fatigue, or widespread muscle aches. If you do choose to exercise when you're sick, reduce the intensity and length of your workout. Exercising at your normal intensity when you have more than a simple cold puts you at risk for a more serious illness.

Let your body be your guide. If you have a cold and feel miserable, take a break. Scaling back or taking a few days off from exercise when you're sick shouldn't affect your performance. Resume your normal workout routine gradually as you begin to feel better.

# Calcium

The role of calcium in our bodies, and the best sources of obtaining that calcium, are somewhat controversial. We need calcium to maintain our health, such as helping to improve osteoporosis, building and maintaining bones and teeth, the regulation of heart rhythm, the transmission of nerve impulses, and blood clotting. There is some question as to whether calcium from food or supplements can contribute to heart disease. At this time it appears not to do so.

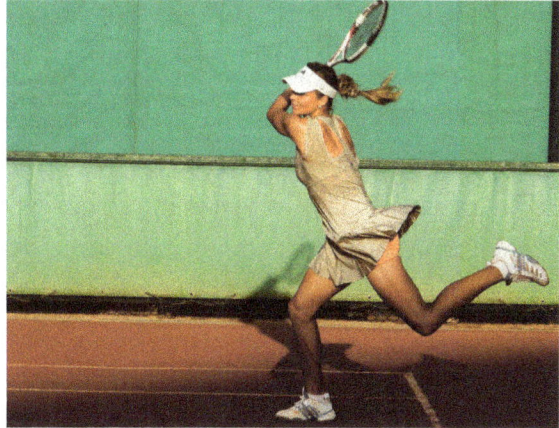

Our bodies obtain the calcium we need from several sources. The main and most important one is from food, such as canned sardines, plain low fat yogurt, calcium fortified rice or soy milk, tofu, and canned salmon. Another source is from calcium supplements often combined with vitamin D. Lastly are the dairy products which have a high concentration per serving of highly absorbable calcium. The pro milk/dairy supporters believe that increased calcium, as found in dairy products, will help to prevent osteoporosis, which now causes more than 1.5 million fractures, with some 300,000 broken hips a year.

In the U.S. milk is usually thought as one of the best sources of calcium. However, after early childhood, there may be more downsides to milk (dairy) consumption such as:

- Lactose intolerance causing abdominal cramping, nausea, vomiting, and diarrhea

- High saturated fat content possibly leading to heart disease

- Possible increased risk of ovarian and prostate cancer

Ninety-nine percent of the body's calcium is stored in our bones. With enough physical activity and normal calcium levels, our bodies build strong bones until about age 30, after which bones  will begin to weaken rather than strengthen. If the calcium level in our bodies gets low, calcium can be "borrowed" from the bones and paid back later when calcium levels return to normal.

Osteoporosis or "porous bones" is a weakening of bones as we age despite normal calcium levels. This has been shown to possibly increase the risk of fractures. More women than men are affected by this condition. This loss of bone with aging can result from a number of factors such as lower levels of the hormones, estrogen in women and testosterone in men, from genetic factors, physical inactivity, and a variety of diseases.

Preventing osteoporosis is dependent on two things: Making the strongest, densest bones before age 30 and limiting bone loss as we age.

Things we can do to limit osteoporosis are:

- Consuming enough calcium to prevent it from being taken from the bones
- Getting enough weight bearing exercise such as walking or running
- Getting adequate vitamin D through diet, supplements, or exposure to the sun
- Consuming adequate green vegetables, fish, meat, and eggs

Vitamin D plays a critical role for bone health. If the calcium level in our blood lowers, vitamin D can act to absorb more calcium from our intestines and also to minimize calcium loss from the kidneys.

Vitamin D sources include: natural sunlight on our skin, fatty fish, foods fortified with vitamin D, and cheese.

The bottom line is that preventing osteoporosis probably goes a long way in preventing fractures.

# Coffee and Health

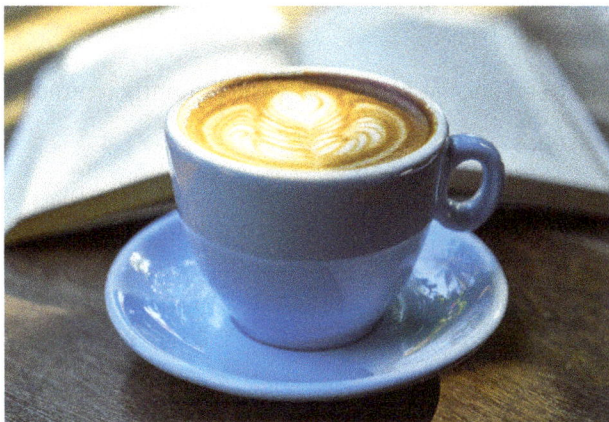

I remember growing up and hearing warnings about consuming too much coffee, because it was possibly related to health problems. Well, my fellow java drinkers, the tide seems to be changing. The results of new studies are coming out showing that coffee consumption, especially in larger quantities, such as 4-6 cups a day, appears to have a beneficial effect on a number of health problems.

It's been estimated that there are more than 1,000 different chemicals found in a cup of coffee. Many of these chemicals are called antioxidants. These are substances that, when floating around the blood stream, can prevent or at least slow damage to many types of cells in our bodies. Although fruits and vegetables are also high in antioxidants, coffee is the main source for most Americans. Some could argue that there must be potentially harmful chemicals found in coffee as well, but so far the benefits of the brew seem to outweigh the risks.

Caffeine is actually a drug and not a nutrient required for good health, as are vitamins and minerals. It is actually a mild stimulant resembling the more potent stimulants, such as cocaine and amphetamine. Its positive effects are related to stimulating the brain and boosting the strength of muscle contractions.

Caffeine does have some short term undesirable side effects, such as raising the blood pressure and causing blood vessels to stiffen. Those with high blood pressure should limit their coffee intake. Young people, who are now drinking highly caffeinated "energy" drinks ought to limit or avoid caffeine, because it is reported that it may weaken developing bones.

Some diseases that have been shown to  occur less frequently from coffee consumption are:

- Alzheimer's disease
- Parkinson's disease
- Certain cancers
- Diabetes
- Liver disease
- Stroke

To those of us who enjoy our cup of joe, continue to do so.  For those who don't, there are many other ways to keep healthy.

# Probiotics

Probiotics are microbes (bacteria) that are believed to provide health benefits when consumed, and can be found in certain foods or supplements that contain these good microbes.

Let's consider the human lower intestinal tract, which is home to some 100 trillion microbes. This is ten times the total number of cells that make up the entire human body. These microbes are considered "good bacteria" and help to digest food, fight some harmful bacteria, and according to some research, may help boost the immune system.

An imbalance of good and bad bacteria in your intestines can make you sick. The most common problem from this imbalance comes when we take antibiotics, which can kill the good intestinal bacteria leading to diseases that cause diarrhea. It's fairly common to have an episode of diarrhea during or after taking an antibiotic. Recent studies have shown a significant decrease of antibiotic associated diarrhea when taking probiotics during and up to a week after taking antibiotics. For greatest effectiveness, do not take probiotics within two hours of taking an antibiotic.

Probiotics may also help traveler's diarrhea, as well as diarrhea caused by the common "stomach flu."

Some other health related conditions have been thought to also be helped by taking probiotics. However, there are few good scientific studies to substantiate these claims. Some of these conditions are:
- Ulcerative colitis and Crohn's disease
- Celiac disease and lactose intolerance
- Constipation and irritable bowel syndrome
- Bacterial vaginal infections

Probiotics are thought to be generally safe for anyone, but due to a rare risk of infection, those with a known immune deficiency or anyone being treated for cancer should avoid them.

Some foods also contain probiotics including yogurt, a fermented dairy drink called Kefir, and some fermented vegetables, such as sauerkraut and pickles. While they may contain probiotics, there's no guarantee that they have them in the amount or type that may have health benefits. Only dietary supplements containing probiotics have been tested and may be helpful.

Most supplements contain freeze dried bacteria which come alive in your digestive system. These products can be found at most drug stores, supermarkets, heath food stores, and online. They come as tablets, capsules, or as a powder.

You need to look for a product that has up to 10 billion colony forming units per day in a single dose. Check for the expiration date for the live bacteria found on the label and follow directions for proper storage.

In summary, although probiotics are touted for treatment of a variety of conditions, the only treatment, which seems to hold up to scientific scrutiny is to help prevent antibiotic associated diarrhea. That said, there appear to be no significant side effects or known health problems for healthy adults who use probiotics for other conditions.

# Salt/Sodium

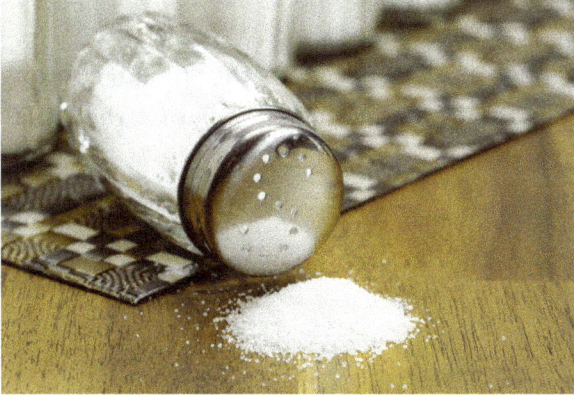

It is frequently reported that the American diet contains too much salt. The reason for this would appear to be that salt greatly enhances the taste of food. We are reported to eat an average of 3,400 mg of salt daily, or the equivalent of 1 1/2 teaspoons. There is some controversy over the daily amount of sodium we should consume, but a reasonable recommendation is a limit of 1,500 mg per day for people with high blood pressure and 2,300 mg daily for everyone else.

We all need a certain amount of sodium found in salt in order to maintain the health of all our cells and organs, as well as to maintain a proper fluid balance within our bodies. In most cases, if we eat too much salt, our kidneys will flush it out. But there are those of us who for whatever reason retain too much sodium, which in turn increases the amount of fluid we retain within our bodies. This will usually manifest as high blood pressure, which can increase the risk of a heart attack or stroke. Other conditions can be adversely affected by too much sodium, such as congestive heart failure and pulmonary edema (a condition where fluid builds up in the lungs making if very difficult to breathe adequately).

Our dietary salt intake comes mostly from the salt shaker, as well as what naturally occurs in foods, and that which is found in processed foods, especially cured or smoked meats. Most processed food we purchase such as canned soup, bread, jarred pasta, and even breakfast cereals can be relatively high in sodium. When shopping for food, look for fresh, frozen (no sauce or seasoning) or low/no salt added packaged goods and canned food.

In place of salt, we can season our food using spices such as rosemary, cumin, basil, dill, or ginger. Garlic or lemon pepper also add a nice non-sodium taste to food, as do flavored vinegars, and  lemon or lime juice.

There are also "salt substitutes" available made from potassium chloride (with very low or no sodium). One main drawback of the substitutes is a bitter aftertaste, which many would not be able to tolerate.

My final advice is to try to eat fresh food as much as possible, check the sodium content on all labels of purchased processed food, keep total daily amount of sodium in the 2,000 mg. range, and keep your hands off of the salt shaker.

# Vitamin D

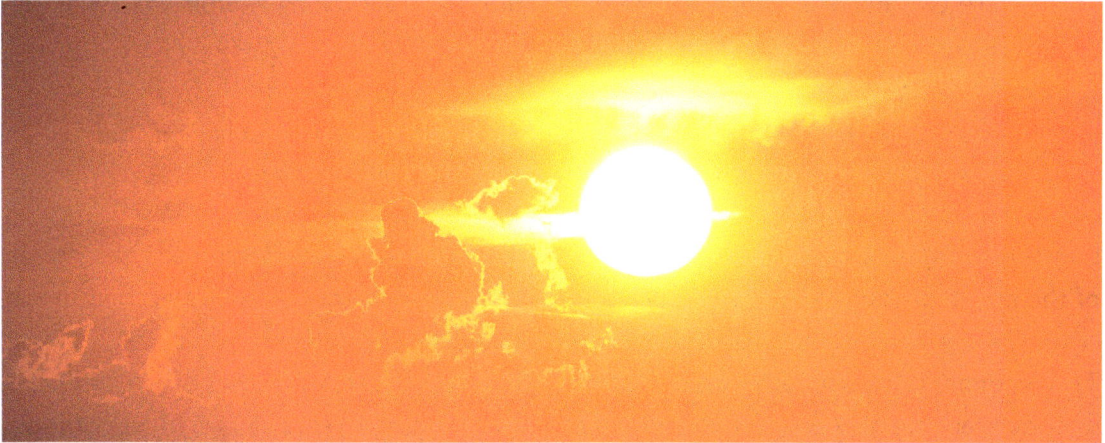

A vitamin is an organic substance essential in small quantities to normal metabolism. It is found naturally in various foods, but it can also be produced artificially. A lack of vitamins can cause certain diseases.

Vitamin D is the only nutrient the human body makes itself. Ultraviolet rays from sun exposure interact with a chemical in the skin to form an inactive version of vitamin D, which is then converted in the liver and kidneys into an active version useful to our bodies.

Because people have been warned to wear sunscreen and to limit sun exposure, we might not be able to manufacture enough of this vitamin on our own and may need to look for other sources.

Vitamin D can be found in a limited number of foods, including fatty fish, fish liver oils, liver, and egg yolks. Commercial milk products, breakfast cereals, and juices are often fortified with low levels of vitamin D. People don't usually eat enough of these foods to consistently cover their daily vitamin D requirements.

The primary benefits of vitamin D for our bodies are these:

- Bone health: Vitamin D helps the body absorb calcium and phosphorus, which are two minerals needed for strong bones. People taking vitamin D have a lower risk of bone fractures and also have been found to have a lower chance of falling.

- Brain function: People with higher blood levels of vitamin D have higher cognitive performance, including memory and thinking skills.

Low levels of vitamin D, by contrast, have been associated with some increased risks: cancer of the colon, breast and prostate, arthritis, diabetes, and infections such as tuberculosis.

The recommended daily allowance (RDA) is 600 IU for those 1-70 years of age and pregnant or breastfeeding women, and 800 IU for those over 71 years of age. Most common multivitamins contain 400 IU. Momentum is building within the medical community to increase the daily recommended dose to at least 800 to 1,000 IU. From what I can tell, this is a reasonable recommendation. The higher level should help to strengthen bones and muscles and hopefully prevent a variety of diseases, such as those I have mentioned.

## Abdominal Pain

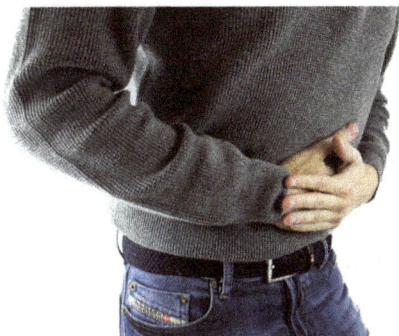

All of us at one time or another have experienced abdominal pain. It is one of the most common complaints seen in emergency rooms. Most of the time it is not caused by a serious medical problem, but when it is serious it can be life threatening. In this article I'd like to differentiate between mild pain symptoms and more serious symptoms that would cause you to seek urgent medical care.

There are an abundant number of causes of abdominal pain too numerous to mention in this article, but there are many signs and symptoms of abdominal pain of which you should be aware.

What are the most common causes of abdominal pain?

- Indigestion, constipation, ulcers, and gas
- Stomach flu and food poisoning
- Food allergies and lactose intolerance
- Gallstones and kidney stones
- Urinary tract infections, pelvic infections, ovarian disease, endometriosis, and menstrual cramps

More serious causes include:

- Aneurysm (swelling with possible rupture) of the aorta
- Decreased blood supply to the intestines (ischemic bowel)
- Appendicitis, diverticulitis, and cholecystitis, (infections of the appendix, the colon, and the gall bladder respectively)
- Bowel blockage (obstruction)

- Cancer of any of the intra-abdominal organs, especially of stomach, colon, or liver
- Pancreatitis (inflammation of the pancreas)
- Pneumonia
- Heart attack

Seek immediate medical help or call 911 for abdominal pain that involves:

- Severe sudden abdominal pain
- Vomiting blood, having blood in your stool, or if your stool appears tar colored
- Tenderness over your abdomen, or if it feels rigid when you touch it
- Pregnancy either confirmed or suspected
- A recent injury to your abdomen
- Pain and difficulty breathing
- Mild abdominal pain that does not improve within 24-48 hours, or becomes more severe or frequent, especially if occurring with vomiting
- Diarrhea for more than several days, especially with fever or blood
- Fever over 100°F (37.7°C) with your pain

I have tried to simplify the complex subject of abdominal pain. Obviously this is not all inclusive, but my goal has been to have you understand those symptoms that should prompt immediate medical attention.

# Leg Cramps

Most of us have at one time or another had a nocturnal leg cramp. Some individuals suffer frequently from them. Almost anyone can experience cramps, but they are more common in the elderly. Although they are technically harmless, they can be quite debilitating sometimes lasting 15 minutes or more. Most cramps have no obvious underlying cause.

It is believed that cramps may be associated with dehydration, prolonged sitting, or a deficiency of certain electrolytes, such as magnesium, potassium, or calcium. Some medications have also been implicated, including diuretics, oral contraceptives, and beta blockers. Cramps have also been related to conditions, such as pregnancy, diabetes, and thyroid disorders.

There is weak evidence that B-complex vitamins and magnesium supplements may help to prevent cramps. Most other food and natural supplements have not been found to be helpful.

What to do for a leg cramp? First try massaging the cramped muscle. Next, try flexing your feet by bringing your toes up toward your knees. Try applying either hot or cold compresses directly to the painful muscle. Lastly, if you're not in too much pain, try to get up and walk around.

Here are some suggestions for reducing the frequency of cramps:
- Maintain adequate hydration by drinking plenty of water throughout the day. This especially important if you've been working out and/or sweating.
- Massage and stretch your calf muscles before retiring. For stretching, try standing two or three feet from a wall with one foot forward. Lean forward with forearms up against the wall, keeping rear knee straight with the rear heel flat on the floor. Hold for 20-30 seconds then switch legs and repeat.
- Loosen or untuck bedcovers and sheets at foot of bed in order to give your feet plenty of room.

- Avoid high heel shoes, as well as completely flat shoes. Wear shoes with good support.

In the past, quinine was traditionally used as a treatment for leg cramps, but due to its dangerous side effects, it is no longer recommended. In fact quinine products are no longer sold over the counter.

If you have tried all the above suggestions and still suffer from nocturnal leg cramps, see your doctor.

# Migraine Headache

Migraine headaches are common in our population, affecting some 17% of all women and 6% of men. These headaches are brought about by changes in a body chemical called serotonin, which when levels are high, can cause blood vessels to shrink. When levels are low, blood vessels dilate, which is what causes the headache.

There are typically two types of migraines. One is associated with an aura, which occurs before the headache and produces symptoms of bright flashing colored lights, blurry vision, and unusual sensations in your body. Auras often last 15 to 20 minutes and then are usually (but not always) followed by a headache. The other type of migraine causes only the headache without an aura.

The typical migraine headache can be quite severe and is often on only one side of the head, but occasionally is on both sides. The quality of pain can be either steady or throbbing. Other accompanying symptoms can include nausea, vomiting, and sensitivity to light. These headaches may occur only once or twice a year or as often as daily. Migraines can last from several hours to more than 72 hours.

Certain foods can trigger migraine, such as:

- Aged cheese
- Chocolate
- Pickled foods
- Alcoholic beverages

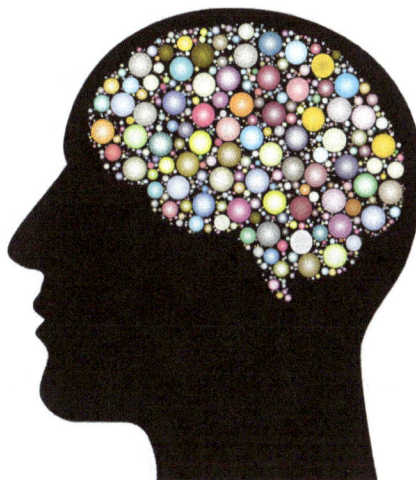

Other migraine triggers:
- Bright lights, loud noises
- Fatigue, stress
- Intense physical activity
- Menstrual periods, birth control pills

There are two types of migraine treatment. One type is the use of either over the counter pain medications such as ibuprofen (Advil), naproxen (Aleve), or acetaminophen (Tylenol) or with prescription migraine medication, which may be prescribed by your doctor. Treatment should be started as soon as the pain begins. If these medications have been used but are not effective in relieving the pain, a visit to your doctor may be necessary.

Several years ago the FDA approved the use of Botox injections to help relieve migraine pain when the more traditional treatment has failed.

Nontraditional therapies may also help in treating chronic headache pain such as:
- Acupuncture
- Massage
- Herbs - feverfew and butterbur
- Minerals- magnesium sulfate supplements
- Vitamins- Riboflavin (vitamin B-2)

Symptoms of headaches more serious than migraine and needing prompt medical attention are:
- A severe sudden headache like a "thunderclap"
- Headache with stiff neck, fever, rash, confusion
- Headache after a head injury
- New headache pain if you're older than 50

# Peripheral Neuropathy

Peripheral neuropathy is caused by damage to certain nerves mostly the sensory nerves which deal with touch, pain, and heat. Most of the time the problem starts in the fingers and toes and can worsen to include the feet, legs, and hands.

Causes of peripheral neuropathy include:
- Diabetes (the most common cause)
- Chemotherapy
- Alcoholism
- Vitamin deficiencies

The most common symptoms are:
- Pain, burning or tingling of fingers, toes, hands, and feet
- Muscle weakness and balance problems
- Loss of sensation to touch
- Difficulty using fingers, such as buttoning one's clothing

Measures that may help relieve the symptoms of neuropathy:
- Acupuncture, massage, physical therapy, and reflexology
- Relaxation therapy
- Prescribed medications, such as pain medicine, lidocaine patches, capsaicin cream, anti-depressant, and anti-seizure medications
- Vitamins and supplements, such as vitamins B1, B6, B12 and alpha lipoic acid. Check with your doctor for proper doses and any other treatment options

How to take care of yourself:
- Because neuropathy can cause poor balance, remove throw rugs and clear up any clutter

- Put grab bars near shower, bathtub, or toilet
- Protect your hands and feet where sensation is decreased and be aware of contact with very hot or cold temperatures
- Don't drink alcohol
- Check hands and feet for cuts, scrapes, burns, or any other signs of injury

If you think you are having any of the symptoms of neuropathy, see your doctor for evaluation and suggested treatment.

# Sciatica

Sciatica is a symptom manifested by pain and often a "pins and needles" sensation running through the buttock and down one's leg all the way to the toes. The pain may be worse when you sit, sneeze or cough, and can occur suddenly, although it usually has a more gradual onset.

Causes of sciatica include:

- A herniated disc — "ruptured or slipped disc" is the most common cause and occurs from the pressure of a bulging disc from between 2 back bones, thus putting pressure on nearby nerve roots

- Spinal stenosis — Results from age related narrowing of the spinal canal putting pressure on sciatic spinal nerve roots

- Spondylolisthesis — Slippage of one vertebral bone so as to make it out of line with the one above it, narrowing the opening through which the nerve exits

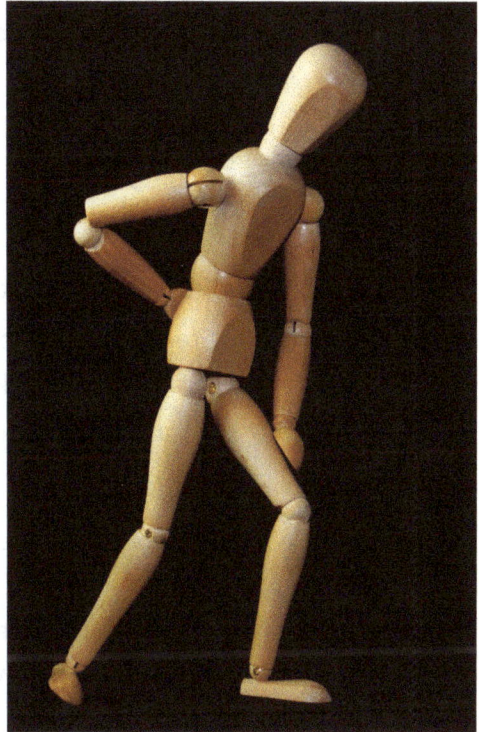

Sciatica is usually diagnosed by your doctor providing you with a good history and physical exam. Depending on what your doctor finds, further testing may be done including:

- A plain X-ray of the back.

- An MRI, which can be diagnostically extremely helpful when necessary. It is very expensive and usually only needed for severe symptoms or for symptoms not improving in a timely manner.

- Nerve conduction studies to determine how well electrical impulses travel through the sciatic nerve

Treatment usually includes limited physical rest, the use of medications to control pain when necessary, and developing a customized physical therapy program.

If pain persists or worsens, spinal injections using cortisone to the involved area can be helpful.

Ultimately surgery can be performed for those who have had no improvement by any other means.

Reducing one's risk of developing sciatica may include:

- Proper lifting techniques – lifting by keeping your back straight bringing yourself upright using your hips, legs, and knees
- Exercising regularly to strengthen your back and abdominal muscles
- Avoid sitting for long periods
- Using good posture at all times

Sciatic pain usually goes away with time and conservative treatment often within the first 6 weeks. Up to 90 percent of people with sciatica will improve without surgery.

See your doctor for any questions and concerns.

# Shoulder Pain

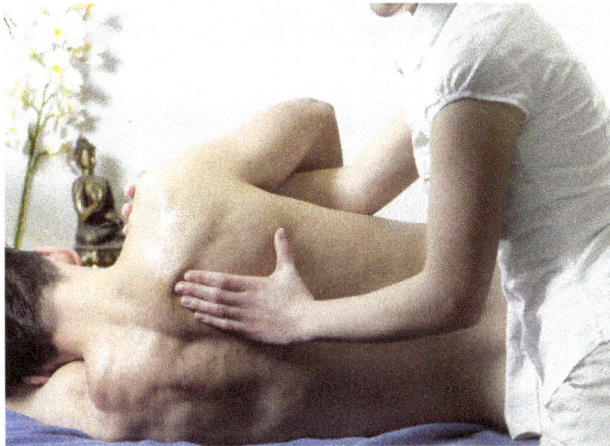

Shoulder pain is common in older adults affecting some 30 % of adult Americans. The shoulder joint is essentially made up of three bones: the upper arm bone (humerus), the shoulder blade (scapula), and the collar bone (clavicle). The uppermost part of the humerus fits into a socket in the shoulder blade and is surrounded by supporting tendons and muscles referred to as the rotator cuff. The rotator cuff helps to provide shoulder motion and stability.

Causes of shoulder pain include:

**Impingement** — When the top of the shoulder blade puts pressure on the underlying soft tissues as the arm is lifted away from the body. This leads to inflammation and pain, and over time can lead to a rotator cuff tear and eventual surgery.

**Bursitis/Tendonitis** — Inflammation of the tissues surrounding the shoulder joint often leading to rotator cuff pain.

**Arthritis** — This is from inflammation of the shoulder joint due to "chronic wear and tear." This usually becomes prominent during middle age and is manifested by swelling, pain, and stiffness. It is often related to sports or work injuries and chronic wear and tear.

**Injury** — Prior fracture or dislocation can lead to chronic shoulder pain.

After a history and physical exam from your doctor, he/she will likely order an imaging study such as a plain X-ray, a MRI, or a CT scan.

Treatment usually involves rest, modifying activities, and physical therapy. Avoiding activities that cause the pain is an obvious must. Medications to relieve pain and inflammation, and injections, are also treatments your doctor may use.

Surgery may eventually be necessary, but some 90% of those with shoulder pain will respond to simple non surgical treatment as mentioned above.

If your shoulder joint aches for more than a few weeks, it's probably time to see your doctor for evaluation and treatment.

## Father's Day

DOCTORS ARE FATHERS TOO

Happy Father's Day to my grandfather, Norman Hollenbeck, M.D., and to my father, Stanley Hollenbeck, M.D. You both were the inspiration that led me to my chosen career of medicine. How proud I felt when I graduated from the same medical school both of you attended and graduated.

Grandpa, because of your untimely death, I never really knew you, but I grew up hearing stories about your life. The wife you left behind, my wonderful Grandma Lillian Hollenbeck, told me all about you. It's amazing to think of the days of doctors making house calls, and you even did it in a horse and buggy. What was it like practicing medicine without CAT scans, antibiotics, comprehensive blood tests, intensive care units, paramedics, and all the things we take for granted today? You made life-and-death decisions without the use of medical specialists, computers, X-rays, or blood tests.

When people had no ability to pay you for your services, you accepted chickens and vegetables. Some of your patients couldn't even afford that. You delivered babies, and continued treating them as they grew older. You were the only doctor most of your patients ever knew.

My favorite story about you was when you delivered a baby at someone's home, which was the custom then. Apparently, after the baby was born, the mother hemorrhaged and lost a lot of blood. She was in danger of dying, and there was no time to get to the hospital (there weren't emergency rooms then, anyhow). So, you called one of your medical colleagues, and right there in the patient's bed, you two doctors hooked up an IV line from your arm directly into her bloodstream. You gave your very own blood to save her life. She lived, but you became very anemic and had to recuperate for several months. That's a story that's almost too hard to believe, except that Grandma gave me a copy of the article from the local newspaper, which I proudly possess. You died way too young, but you left an incredible legacy for my father and me to follow.

Dad, I grew up and remember hearing so often from people how you were one of the greatest high school football players to come out of the city of Milwaukee. Octogenarians today in Milwaukee still remember your football fame. How sad that during your last high school football game, you sustained a severe knee injury that prevented you from pursuing the professional career that everyone expected of you.

So you chose the medical career of your father. Shortly after you set up your family practice and joined the Wisconsin National Guard, World War II broke out and you were called up to active service. You were part of the 32nd Red Arrow Division of the US Army. After a quick basic training, you and your comrades were sent to Buna, New Guinea, in the South Pacific. There you were the commander of the 14th Portable Surgical Hospital, which was the forerunner of the MASH unit, which became so well known in the Korean War. You kept a diary, which I now possess, that describes your daily life on the front line. You and your crew operated in a hot, steamy lantern-lit canvas tent, trying to patch together the wounds of the brave young soldiers who were engaged with an enemy literally within several hundred yards from your hospital tent. You saw more horrible things in that war than I could ever imagine. I know you carried those memories with you the rest of your life. You were a true hero, and I have in its original frame the Silver Star you so deservedly won for gallantry in action.

You came back from the war (thank God) and continued your very successful general medical practice. As a young boy, I was always so proud being with you, because everywhere we went, you were constantly recognized by your patients and greeted with a hearty, "Hi Doc, how ya doin." I loved going on house calls with you and making Sunday morning hospital rounds. I remember that almost anytime you took me somewhere, whether it was to a Milwaukee Braves baseball game or a Green Bay Packers football game, you would be paged to go to the hospital. You received countless phone calls from patients day and night, and you took only two weeks of vacation a year. But I knew from early on that after watching and helping you treat patients in your office (at that time downstairs in our home) that I wanted to be just like you.

So, Grandpa and Dad, Happy Father's day, and thanks for the inspiration to pursue the wonderful career I have chosen.

# Veteran's Day

November 11 is Veterans Day. Although I never had to serve in the military, I honor those who did. I especially have the highest regard for those who actually saw combat and put their lives on the line for me and my country. To you ladies and gentlemen, I give my deepest thanks.

Today I'd like to honor my favorite veteran, my late father, Stanley Hollenbeck, M.D. Dad was born in 1911, in Milwaukee Wisconsin, where I was also born and raised. He graduated from Marquette University School of Medicine in 1936, and began a private practice. Around that same time he joined the Wisconsin National Guard.

With the onset of WW II, his regiment became part of the Army's 32nd Infantry Division, which was sent to Australia in May of 1942. Dad left behind his new medical practice, his wife, and newborn son, my brother, Stan Jr. I can't imagine how Dad felt about leaving his comfortable life behind, especially not knowing what he would be facing as he would be thrust into the escalating war with Japan in the South Pacific.

Dad was the commanding officer of the 14th Portable Surgical Hospital, one of the army's first M.A.S.H. units, which were later popularized by Alan Alda in the TV hit series "M.A.S.H." Dad and his crew were sent to the north coast of New Guinea near a small village called Buna, where the enemy was deeply entrenched. His unit's bulky, hot, humid hospital tent was set up less than 1,000 yards from the front line where hand to hand combat was taking place.

Health conditions for the troops were among the worst in the world. The mosquitoes and flies were horrific. Almost all soldiers, including Dad, suffered bouts of malaria. Everyone had recurrent dysentery. There were also scrub typhus, dengue fever, hookworm, yaws, and countless cases of "fever of unknown origin." Troops suffered from depression and severe battle fatigue caused by the relentless hot, humid, rainy weather, the jungle, and inadequate food. For every two men who were battle casualties, five were out of action from fever and illness.

Dad and his crew often operated day and night on the young wounded soldiers, which took place in a large canvas tent by lantern light. Temperatures inside the tent could reach up to 120 degrees. All of this was done under frequent machine gun strafing and bombing by enemy fighter planes, as well as the constant threat of being overrun by enemy troops.

Dad kept a daily diary of his life in New Guinea, which was later published by his VFW group in Milwaukee. Here is an excerpt from that diary: "On November 16, 1942, a five boat convoy bringing desperately needed ammunition, food and medical supplies to the troops was attacked by enemy aircraft setting all the vessels ablaze". Dad and his crew witnessed the event from the shore.

From his diary he further states: "I grabbed my medical kit, forded the river and started up the beach. I could see the boats burning fiercely as night began to fall. I was frightened to death not knowing exactly where the enemy troops would be as I walked along the jungle's edge. I continued up the beach, checked on survivors and rendered first aid. I had the more seriously injured sent back to our hospital tent. I hurried back to get ready to operate on the wounded. We operated all night long on the men, mostly with abdominal wounds, sewing up the bullet holes in their intestines, besides treating other serious wounds. We finally finished, getting to bed at 4:30 AM."

From October 1942 through February 1943, Dad remained just behind the front line, operating and treating wounds on countless injured soldiers. Lives were lost, but many more were saved due to the efforts of Dad and his crew. In February 1943, the 14th Portable Surgical Hospital was awarded the Distinguished Unit of Citation, and several individual members of the unit, including my father, received the Silver Star medal for gallantry in action. He also received the rank of lieutenant colonel.

Dad told me that he and his fellow soldiers were willing to put their lives on the line, believing that a victory would end all wars, and that their children would never have to do the same. Unfortunately, such a dream was not to come true. Sons and daughters are still sent to battle.

To you Dad, of whom I am so very proud, and to all the other brave veterans living and dead, I salute you, and I honor you.

# Anxiety

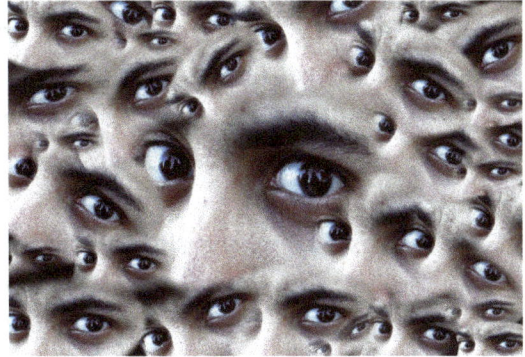

We live in anxious times. The media brings us news of a poor economy, joblessness, people losing homes, international problems, high crime rates, etc. In addition, there are our own personal issues to deal with, such as poor health, relationship difficulties, financial problems, and high pressure jobs. Even every day annoyances stress us out, such as being stuck in traffic, computer problems, and too many appointments, and obligations.

Over 40 million people suffer from anxiety. It can begin in childhood, but most commonly affects the middle aged, and even the elderly. Twice as many women as men have anxiety. Other similar disorders include social phobias, post-traumatic stress disorder, panic disorder, and obsessive-compulsive disorder.

Some of the more common manifestations of anxiety are:

- Constant worrying and obsessing over big or small problems
- Feeling of impending doom or worthlessness
- Fatigue or trouble sleeping
- Restlessness and feeling uptight
- Difficulty concentrating and irritability
- Sweating, nausea, vomiting, shortness of breath, and rapid heart rate

When being evaluated by your doctor for anxiety, physical causes such as thyroid problems, heart or lung disease, and even dietary problems need to be ruled out. Once this is done there are several options for treatment including:

**Psychotherapy** – This involves working with a trained therapist focusing on working out underlying life stresses, concerns, and making behavior changes. This may be done through cognitive behavioral therapy, which is one of the more common types of psychotherapy. It involves learning to identify unhealthy negative beliefs and behaviors that contribute to anxiety, and teaches how to replace them with positive healthy beliefs. These treatments can give us the tools necessary to deal with our responses to life's many problems, and to help one gain control, especially by changing the way we respond to situations.

**Medications** — For the short term, there are benzodiazepines, such as Xanax and Ativan. These can work quickly and effectively, but can be habit forming. For the longer term, antidepressants, such as Zoloft or Celexa can be used. Close medical supervision is important for drug therapy.

**Life style and home remedies —**

- Exercise
- Healthy diet
- Avoid alcohol
- Relaxation techniques such as yoga and meditation
- Adequate sleep

If you think you suffer from anxiety, see your doctor. With evaluation and a personalized treatment plan, your anxiety can be brought under control.

# Depression

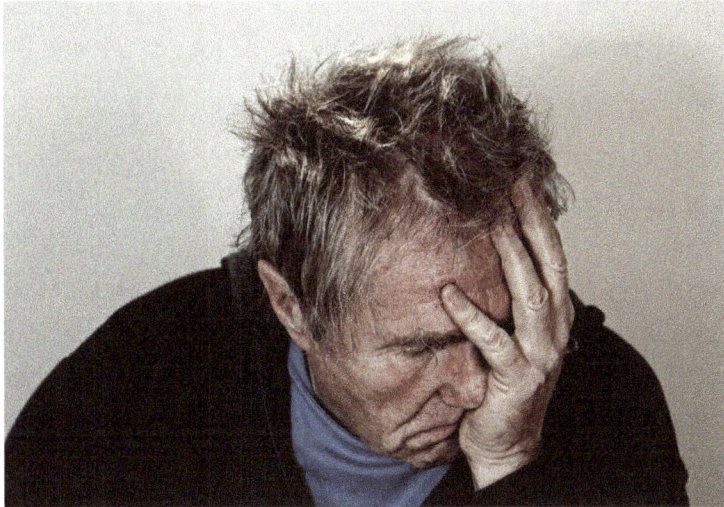

Depression is a true medical illness, similar to having diabetes or high blood pressure. It's not a weakness, having the blues, or something you can just snap out of. Fortunately, like most illnesses, depression is treatable through medication and psychotherapy.

Common symptoms of depression include:

- Feeling sad, unhappy, irritable, or frustrated
- Loss of interest in things that usually bring pleasure
- Feeling worthless or indecisive
- Fatigue, excessive sleeping, or insomnia
- Indecisiveness and decreased concentration
- Thoughts of death, dying, or suicide

Many of us may briefly experience any of the above symptoms, but the person with true depression lives with these symptoms day in and day out.

Some risk factors of depression are:

- Having biological family members with depression, or who have committed suicide

- Experiencing stressful events such as death or loss of a loved one

- Being a woman, especially after a pregnancy

- Having a serious, chronic illness

- Abusing alcohol, drugs, or nicotine

In general, the most effective treatment for depression is a combination of medication and psychotherapy. There are many types of antidepressant drugs available. Finding the right one may take some trial and error. Anti depressant drugs may take several weeks to take effect. If you do experience undesired side effects don't stop taking the medication without consulting your doctor. In many cases you must taper off the drug to avoid withdrawal symptoms.

Psychotherapy is provided by a trained and licensed professional, who can help you to understand your thoughts and behaviors, and allow you to make effective changes. Ideally, this treatment can also provide you with a regained feeling of hope, happiness, and control in your life.

If you, or someone you know, is having suicidal thoughts, help is needed immediately. Here's what needs to be done:

- Contact a family member, friend, or clergy person for assistance

- Call a suicide hotline number

- Seek professional consultation from your doctor or a mental health provider

If you or someone you know is literally on the verge of, or has attempted suicide, call 911 immediately for professional and rapid help.

# Insomnia

It is estimated that about one-third of adults have difficulty sleeping, and are thus sleep deprived. Twenty percent of people get less than six hours of sleep. Adults need seven to nine hours of sleep a night. Any less than this can cause increased stress, a depressed immune system, and can make you cranky and irritable. It also puts one at increased risk for obesity, diabetes, and high blood pressure.

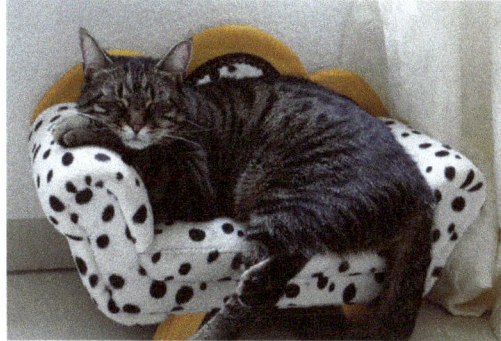

Insomnia becomes more prominent as we age, which is unfortunate because older people still need as much sleep as younger people do. Aging causes a change of sleep patterns leading to a lighter less restful sleep. Decreasing physical and social activity, as well as an increase of chronic health problems, also contribute to less sleep.

Causes of insomnia are:

- Stress

- Anxiety and depression

- Medications, such as heart and blood pressure drugs, steroids, decongestants, and weight loss products

- Caffeine, nicotine, and alcohol

- Medical conditions, such as chronic pain, frequent urination, and sleep apnea

- Change in environment or work schedule

- Eating and drinking too much late in the evening

Non prescription medication remedies should be tried first. These include:

- **Lifestyle changes**. Be consistent with the time you go to bed and when you wake up. Don't nap more than 30 minutes a day, and preferably do it before 3 P.M. Don't linger in bed if you can't sleep. Make your bedroom conducive to sleep by keeping it dark, quiet, and at a comfortable temperature. Limit or avoid caffeine, alcohol, and nicotine. Avoid large late meals. A recent study found that most adults who did aerobic exercise four times a week dramatically improved their sleep.

- **Behavioral therapies**.  Learn relaxation techniques. Limit the time you spend in bed and associate your bed and bedroom only with sleep. See a therapist who specializes in insomnia, someone who may provide a cure for insomnia and not just treat the symptoms with medication.

- **Alternative medicine**. Melatonin and valerian are over the counter supplements, which are marketed as sleep aids. They may be worth a try, however, some studies have shown them to be no more effective than a placebo, and their long term safety record isn't known.

Taking sleeping pills may seem to be an easy solution and prescription medication can be effective in many cases, but should be used for as short a time as possible. Longer term use is thought to contribute to dependence and side effects such as drowsiness, impaired judgment, depression, agitation, and balance problems. Commonly used over the counter sleeping pills are usually antihistamines, which can cause rebound insomnia, as well as some potentially serious side effects, such as daytime drowsiness, dizziness, forgetfulness, and urinary retention. Use these with caution.

If you are not getting the good night rest that you deserve, see your doctor who can help to treat and guide you to having a more restful and satisfying sleep.

## Imaging (X-Rays)

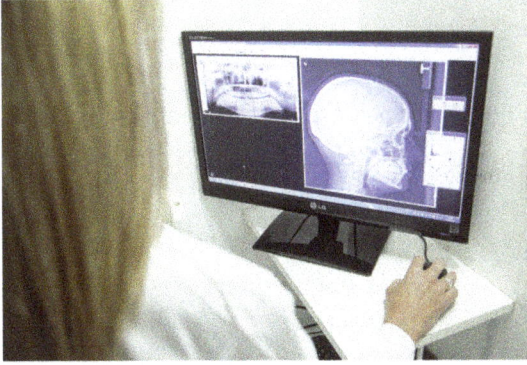

Doctors use diagnostic medical imaging to find out the possible causes of illness, injury, and pain, which helps provide an accurate diagnosis. These images include X-rays, CAT scans, MRIs, and ultrasound.

X-rays were the very first imaging technique and are still the most commonly used today. X-rays use radiation, which produces rays that pass through the body. When striking something dense like bone the image appears white and when going through something hollow like the lungs the image appears black. Muscle and fat appear as shades of gray. Sometimes a dye can be introduced into the body before the X-ray, to enhance the image of certain organs.

X-rays used to be developed on a type of photographic film which needed to be developed and stored. Now the X-ray images can be instantly viewed on a computer screen, eliminating the need for the old film technique. This is a landmark feature, because not only are the digital images immediately available, but they can be sent instantly to another source, such as a consulting physician.

X-rays are still useful for evaluating bones, teeth, the chest (including the lungs and heart), and swallowed opaque items such as coins and most pieces of glass. The digestive tract can be visualized using a dye, such as barium.

Computed axial tomography (CAT/CT) scans use X-rays with computers to produce 360 degree cross sectional views of the body. These views allow the physician to see details of bony structures, chest, heart and lung problems, cancers, and many other internal organs. A typical exam takes 10-30 minutes.

A CAT scanner is much larger and more complex than an X-ray machine. It is a very expensive piece of equipment, and therefore more costly to the patient than an X-ray. In spite of the increased cost, CAT scans can provide the physician with much more information and diagnostic ability than can most X-rays.

CAT scans use substantially more radiation than conventional X-rays, and therefore should be used only when absolutely necessary. Don't hesitate to discuss this with your doctor.

Magnetic resonance imaging (MRI) combines a very powerful magnet along with a computer and radio waves (no radiation exposure), to provide detailed, accurate images of bones, internal organs, soft tissue, and other internal body parts.

Because of the use of the very powerful magnet, patients must be carefully screened to insure that they have nothing metallic in or on the body, such as rings, necklaces, pacemakers, metal implants, and some tattoos.

MRIs often take at least 30 minutes or more, and as with the CAT scan, can take cross-sectional images of the body area being studied. The patient needs to lie completely still inside of a large tube, which may be very difficult for a person with claustrophobia. While inside the tube, the MRI machine makes a very loud knocking sound, usually necessitating wearing ear plugs. The MRI is the most expensive of all the imaging techniques.

Ultrasound uses high frequency sound waves to produce images of structures within our bodies. Like MRIs, it uses no radiation and is very safe. A small hand-held device is pressed against lubricated skin, and is moved around by a trained technician to capture the image. This exam can also be used in a doctor's office or emergency room, making it a very useful diagnostic tool in many circumstances.

# Radiation From Medical Tests

There has been much attention recently, concerning the amount of medical X-ray radiation to which patients are being exposed. As with most medical procedures, X-rays are safe when used with care, especially since in most cases a minimal amount of radiation is used to obtain the needed results.

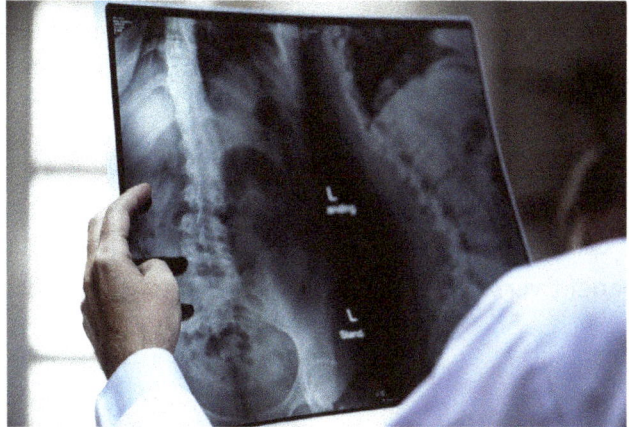

Why worry about radiation exposure? Radiation in sufficient doses can ultimately cause cancer. It is difficult to arrive at any accurate figure of the exact number of cancer cases due to X-ray exposure, although, it is probably fairly low.

The recent concern about radiation exposure is with the newer generation of X-ray exams, especially CT (CAT) scans. About 60 million of these scans are done yearly in the U.S. This computerized type of X-ray exam has revolutionized the ability of a physician to diagnosis many critical diseases and injuries such as appendicitis, stroke, blood clots in the lungs, kidney stones, internal injuries from accidents, heart attacks, and many more serious medical problems. However, these scans expose one to much higher doses of radiation than ordinary X-rays.

Technological advances can help in reducing radiation exposure. Newer scanners may use less radiation, and newer guidelines may allow doctors to use CT scans less often. Attitudes about scanning may need to change as well. Doctors and patients need a heightened level of awareness of the amount of radiation to which one is being exposed.

Another source of concern is the "entire body" scan, which has recently been made popular through direct advertising to the public, and can probably cause more harm than good.

In addition to medical diagnostic radiation, we are all exposed to natural environmental radiation, which comes from cosmic forces such as the sun, rocks, and minerals. You may live in an area with a high exposure to radon gas in your house, which can give you added exposure to radiation. There is also exposure, although very minimal, to man-made factors, such as nuclear weapons testing fallout, industrial sources, luminous watch dials, and smoke detectors.

The bottom line is that you should agree to have a radiation-based medical test when it can improve your health or save your life. Your doctor should discuss with you the benefit versus the risk of any X-ray test that is ordered for you.

# Asthma

It is estimated that over 8 percent of the U.S. population suffers from asthma, and the numbers are rising yearly. This translates into 18 million adults and 7 million children with the disease.

Asthma causes over 3,000 deaths yearly, along with 500,000 hospitalizations, 2 million emergency room visits, and 9 million doctor office visits. Asthma costs the U.S. economy $56 billion per year. This disease has a tremendous financial impact on our families, our nation, and our health care system.

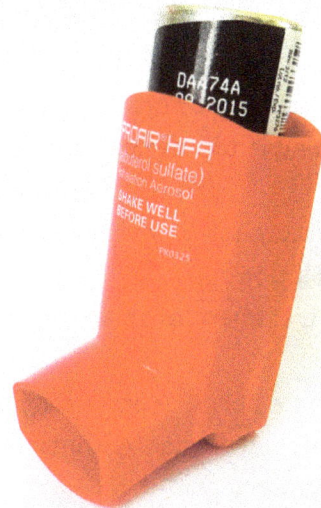

Asthma occurs when the small airways deep in our lung tissue become swollen and narrowed. This makes it difficult for air to pass through these airways, causing the usual symptoms of wheezing and shortness of breath. It can be deadly if not treated promptly and properly.

It is unclear why asthma affects some people and not others. It is probably due to environmental as well as genetic factors.

For some people, asthma symptoms flare up under certain circumstances, such as:

- Allergy induced asthma, triggered by such things as pollen, grasses, pet dander, and dust
- Exercise induced asthma, which is triggered by exercise or exertion
- Occupational asthma from exposure to chemical fumes, dust, or gasses

A number of factors have been identified as increasing one's chance of developing asthma:

- Having a close relative (parent or sibling) with asthma
- Having any other allergic condition, such as hay fever or eczema

- Being overweight or a smoker

- Exposure to second hand smoke or other air borne pollution

Treatment of asthma can be broken down into two categories. First, for quick relief, a drug called albuterol is the mainstay of treating an acute (happening now) attack. This drug is taken by breathing it into the affected lung airways by using either hand held device or a table top device called a nebulizer.

Secondly, for more long-term treatment, inhaled corticosteroids, such as Flovent, have revolutionized the treatment of asthma by helping to prevent attacks and also aiding in the treatment of an acute attack.

I can't emphasize enough how important it is to have an asthma action plan worked out with your doctor. Asthma is an ongoing condition that needs constant monitoring and treatment.

## Bacterial Infections

There are several common bacterial skin infections:

**Impetigo**: This is very contagious, more common in children 2 to 5 years of age, and occurring mostly on the face, especially around the nose and mouth. It can also be found on the arms and legs.

It is caused by the Staphylococcus aureus germ, starting out as small blisters and progressing to a yellow crusty lesion. A child with an open wound or scratch is more susceptible to impetigo, and most people contract the infection from someone else who has it through direct contact or by touching contaminated clothing, bedding, and other objects.

It can be treated with an over the counter ointment called Bactroban. Rarely, for more severe infections, oral antibiotics may be necessary, which you can obtain through your doctor.

**Boils**: These are skin infections usually caused by the Staphylococcus aureus germ that begin in a hair follicle or oil gland. Once the infection begins it may appear as a simple pimple. The area around it becomes red and tender and starts to form a lump as pus begins to develop. As this progresses, it becomes what is called an abscess or furuncle. Several boils grouped together form a more serious infection called a carbuncle.

Treating the beginning boil at home in the early stages involves applying comfortably hot compresses multiple times for 10 to 15 minutes. This may help to draw the pus to the skin surface to get it to drain (rupture) spontaneously. Do not use a needle to "pop" the lesion and do not squeeze it.

If the boil becomes larger (1 to 2 inches), more red, painful, tender, and soft, it probably needs to be drained (lanced) by your doctor. This involves numbing the involved area with a shot of numbing medicine, then making an incision with a scalpel to allow the pus to drain out. This will usually allow the lesion to heal without any further treatment. Keeping the drained boil covered and washing it with soap and water daily, will help to prevent it from spreading to yourself or to those around you.

You can help to prevent boils by:
- Practicing good personal hygiene
- Cleaning and treating minor skin wounds
- Avoiding close contact with anyone else infected with boils

**Cellulitis**: This is a spreading bacterial infection of the skin and tissues immediately under the skin. It is usually caused by the Streptococcus or Staphylococcus germs, which enter the skin through small breaks, such as a scratch. It is frequently found on the legs but can infect any part of the body. Redness, tenderness, pain, chills, and fever are the usual symptoms.

In its earliest stages, comfortably hot compresses and rest  may be the only treatment necessary. However, most cellulitis is cured with antibiotics taken by mouth, as prescribed by your doctor. This should start improving the infection within a few days. For more severe and rapidly progressing infections, hospitalization with IV antibiotics would be necessary.

See your doctor if you have symptoms of these skin conditions.

# Fungal Infections

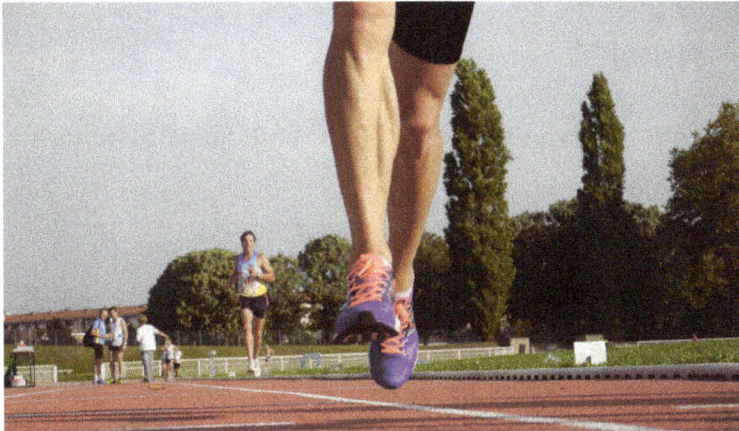

There are several common fungal infections of the skin:

**Athlete's foot**:  is caused by the fungus tinea pedis, usually causing redness, itching, burning, peeling, and blisters. It is found most commonly between the toes but also along the surface of the bottom of the foot.

It is more common in warm, moist environments, such as in shoes, socks, locker rooms, and around swimming pools and showers. It is treated with anti fungal creams or with oral antifungal medication for more severe infections. It can be prevented by wearing sandals in public swimming and showering areas, washing the feet daily with soap and water then drying the skin thoroughly, and by wearing breathable shoes.

**Ringworm**: is caused by the fungus tinea corporis (not by a worm). It can cause red flat lesions often with a central clearing giving it the appearance of a "ring," and can be found just about anywhere on the body. These lesions can range in size from less than an inch to many inches in diameter.

It is spread by direct skin to skin contact from another infected person, from pets, and other contaminated surfaces, especially in a hot and humid environment. Treatment is with an anti fungal cream or with an oral medication for a more extensive rash.

**Jock Itch**: is caused by the *tinea cruris* fungus, and is a rash usually found in the genital region and inner thighs where it likes the warm moist environment. It is mildly contagious. Treatment involves keeping the area clean and dry, changing underwear daily, and using anti fungal creams or sprays.

Common over the counter creams used for all of these fungal infections include:

- Lotrimin, Mycelex
- Lamisil
- Monistat-Derm, Micatin

Six to eight weeks of treatment may be often necessary for a cure. If this doesn't seem to be working effectively, a visit to your doctor may be necessary for stronger prescription treatment.

# Hair Loss

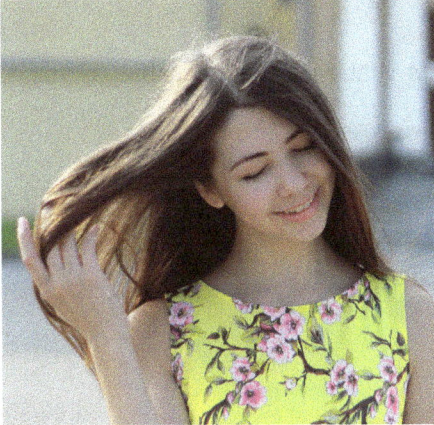

Hair loss is a normal part of aging for men and even for some women. It is estimated that two thirds of men will begin to become bald by the age of 60.

The most common form of baldness, called male or female pattern balding, is often controlled by genetics. It has been commonly believed that baldness was passed down by the mother's genes, but it is now recognized that the father's genes play a role as well.

Women's hair loss pattern is different from that of men, in that women tend to get generalized thinning of the hair rather than distinct balding patterns. Hair loss increases with women's age as it does with men, but about ten percent of premenopausal women will start to lose hair.

There are many other less common causes of balding, including some cancer chemotherapy, severe emotional stress, hormonal changes during pregnancy, severe infections, strict dieting, thyroid disease, certain medications, and some vitamin and nutritional deficiencies.

There is as yet no cure for baldness, but there is an abundance of treatments touted as curing baldness or at least lessening further hair loss. In fact American males collectively spend around one billion dollars a year on these products. Most nonprescription treatments, especially those that are not FDA approved, are worthless in spite of the claims and testimonies.

There are now two approved medicines for treating baldness. Rogaine (Minoxidil and generics) is an over the counter topical solution. It has been shown to be somewhat helpful in halting further hair loss and possibly encouraging new hair growth. It is also the only medication approved to treat female pattern baldness. Both sexes must continue to use this medicine indefinitely. Hair loss starts again when it stops being used.

The other drug, Propecia (Finasteride), is a prescription medication, approved only for men, and taken as a pill by mouth. It also has also been shown to slow or prevent further hair loss.

Both Rogaine and Propecia have potential side effects that make it advisable to speak with your doctor before using either drug.

There are many untrue myths about causes of baldness including:

- Excessive wearing of a hat
- Frequent exposure to sun
- Daily shampooing
- Use of hair spray and gel

Losing some 50 to 100 hairs a day is considered normal. The bottom line is that if you are experiencing what you consider to be hair loss beyond normal, talk to your primary care doctor or dermatologist. Do this before spending a lot hard earned money on worthless treatments.

# Hives

Hives are an outbreak of red blotches on the skin. They can be less than an inch in diameter, to greater than twelve inches, and can be found anywhere on the body. You may not feel them, or they may be intensely itchy. They can often move around or come and go right in front of your eyes. Unlike most other rashes, pressing on an area of a red hive may cause it to blanch white.

Hives are often due to an allergic reaction to foods such as nuts, chocolate, eggs, fresh berries, and milk, to name a few. Medications such as penicillin and sulfa also commonly cause hives. Physical stimulation of the skin from rubbing, scratching, pressure, cold, heat, and even exercise, can cause a hive reaction.

Another condition called angioedema is similar to hives, but involves swelling just beneath the skin, most commonly around the eyes, the lips, and can sometimes involve the hands and feet.

Hives and angioedema are both caused by a release of a chemical called *histamine*, which can leak out of small blood vessels in the skin as a response to an allergic or physical stimulus.

In the short term, hives and angioedema are treated with over the counter antihistamine drugs such as Benadryl, Chlortrimeton, or one of the newer non drowsy drugs, such as Claritin and Allegra. If either hives or angioedema persist (chronic urticaria), then a cortisone drug such as prednisone could be prescribed by your doctor.

In rare cases, hives can be the precursor to a condition called anaphylaxis, a severe allergic reaction that can cause immediate death, such as seen in a person who dies from a bee sting. A person undergoing such a reaction needs an immediate shot of a drug called adrenaline, which can be either self injected by use of an Epi-Pen, or treatment by emergency personnel. The same urgency and treatment goes for severe angioedema, which can cause life threatening swelling around the lips, mouth and throat.

One of the best ways of dealing with hives or urticaria is to avoid known triggering factors, such as certain foods, drugs, or physical stimuli.

For anyone affected by either of these conditions, a referral to an allergist will be necessary for proper diagnosis and treatment options.

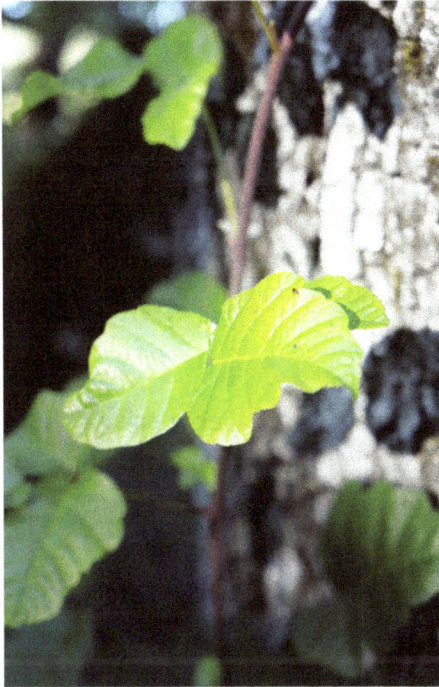

Having treated thousands of cases of poison oak in my career, I'd like to share with you what I've learned about this miserable affliction.

The poison oak plant, which is so prevalent in many locales, contains an oil in its sap called *urushiol*. This oil is found in all parts of the plant; leaves, stems, and roots. Even in extremely minute quantities, it can cause a very severe allergic reaction to our skin. This usually occurs within **24-36** hours after exposure.

Eighty five percent of our population is susceptible to this rash, and a lucky fifteen percent have a natural resistance to it.

You can be exposed to the oil by direct contact with any part of the plant, or by indirect contact with an object such as your own hands, clothing, tools, or anything that may have the urushiol oil on it. There have also been reported cases of smoke from burning poison oak causing either a skin rash or a reaction in the lungs, although I have never seen this in any patient I've treated.

Once you contact the oil, you have only a matter of minutes to wash it off before it will bind to the skin and begin the allergic rash. The best way to remove the oil from the skin is to rinse with lots of water and then wash with soap and water. Most any kind of soap will do. Also, wash any object that may have come in contact with the oil using soap and water, including the clothes you were wearing. And don't forget to do the same to your shoes, tools, and pets. Urushiol oil can remain active on inanimate objects for over a year.

There are a number of over the counter products including Technu and Zanfel, which are to be used on the skin after exposure to poison oak, to remove the oil. I have heard mixed reviews on their effectiveness. For now, I'll stick with water and soap.

Poison oak rash never becomes systemic. It is medically called a "contact dermatitis," and the only place where a rash can develop is where the urushiol oil has contacted the skin. Poison oak rash can affect almost any part of the body. The rash does not spread by touching it even if it is oozing a liquid, although it may seem to when it breaks out on new areas over a number of days. This may happen because the oil absorbs more slowly on thicker skin, such as the forearms, legs or trunk, and faster on thinner skin such as the face and genitals.

Can poison oak rash be prevented before contact with the oil? Some allergy pills or shots have been used with limited success, but in general they are no longer used because of potentially serious side effects.

A poison oak rash will always eventually clear up on its own if one is willing to wait it out. There are an abundance of home remedies to cure poison oak, none of which have been proven to be effective. However, there is effective, proven, and safe medical treatment for those who wish not to suffer for several weeks. Your doctor may prescribe some form of a steroid cream which is stronger and much more effective than over-the-counter cortisone cream. If the rash is more serious and especially involving the face, systemic treatment may be necessary. This involves the use of cortisone pills called prednisone, which is my preferred treatment, or as a steroid shot. Either of these treatments is safe and very effective for most patients. Your doctor will help to determine the best treatment for your particular condition.

The bottom line is that you should avoid contact with poison oak, wash your skin and clothing as soon as possible if you do come in contact, and see your doctor for effective medical treatment if symptoms persist or worsen.

# Summer Skin Injuries

Summer activities bring increased chance of injury to our skin. I would like to describe several common wounds, how to treat them at home and when to seek professional medical treatment.

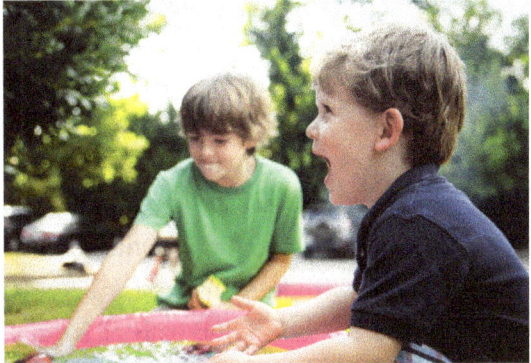

**Abrasions** are scrapes to the skin usually from falling or brushing up against a hard surface. This wound is often quite painful, but rarely serious. The abrasion should be washed with a clean wash rag using water and soap. Most any soap works well with plain hand soap being the most available. Regular tap water works just fine. Gentle scrubbing is all that's necessary unless the wound is contaminated with dirt, such as a "road burn" from falling off of a bicycle. In this case, more vigorous scrubbing may be necessary to remove the contaminant. After cleansing the wound it should be dried off with a clean dry towel, and an antibiotic ointment such as Polysporin or Bacitracin (or even plain petroleum jelly) should be applied directly over the wound. It has been proven that a moist wound heals faster than a dry one. The wound may then be covered with a Band-Aid or other sterile non-stick dressing, such as Adaptic. One may bathe as usual with a new dressing applied after each bath. This should be done daily until the wound has formed a dry scab. At such a time the wound will continue to heal with no further treatment. Medical care should be sought if the abrasion is too painful or too contaminated with dirt to adequately clean.

**Lacerations** are cuts to the skin. Unlike an abrasion a laceration will usually penetrate all layers of the skin and will most often necessitate a trip to your health care provider. One of the most common fears a person has who has cut themselves is that of severe bleeding. Indeed, this is a major concern with certain lacerations. I want to emphasize that almost all laceration bleeding can be controlled by pressure. This can be done by applying firm pressure directly over the wound, preferably with some type of a clean cloth-like material, but using one's bare hand is acceptable if absolutely necessary. This should be continued until professional medical treatment is available. Tourniquets applied to an arm or leg should be used as a last resort, only if direct pressure can't stop the bleeding. The use of tourniquets when not appropriate can do more harm than good.

A small laceration that is not bleeding and has its edges close together can usually be treated at home by the same process described above for abrasions: soap, water, ointment, and Band-Aid. However, most common lacerations either bleed persistently or have wound edges that have separated. These will usually need professional medical treatment, which will involve closure of the wound. This will stop the bleeding and will allow the wound to heal faster with less chance for a secondary infection. Most laceration repair is done using sutures [stitches]. Virtually all sutures applied to the outside of the skin will need to be removed after a certain amount of time. Sutures that dissolve are used under the skin with deeper lacerations. We now have the option of closing some lacerations using a type of liquid super glue. To qualify for this method, a laceration shouldn't be too long, should not be actively bleeding, and not over a joint such as a knee or knuckle. Lacerations to the face are the best candidates for glue closure. The advantage of using glue is that no painful shots are given and there is no need to return for suture removal. The amount of scarring or the chance of infection is no different between the use of sutures versus glue.

If you have sustained one of the above mentioned injuries and you have not had a tetanus shot in the past 10 years and you are unsure of the severity or proper treatment of the wound, you should seek professional medical care.

# Sun Protection

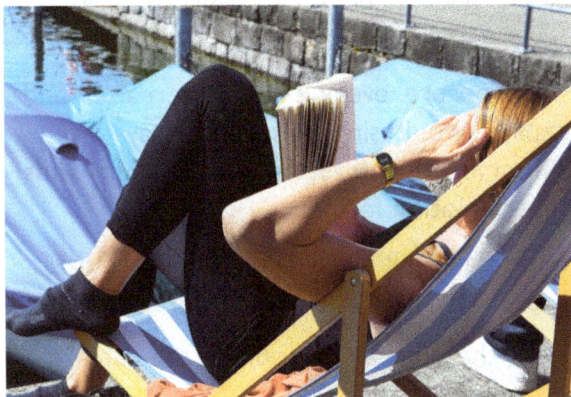

I'd like to make my annual plea for the liberal use of a sunscreen to protect all of us, young and old, from the damaging effects of the sun. Please understand that the "healthy" bronze tan color that many people seek is actually how the skin demonstrates that it has been damaged by the sun.

The sun produces two types of invisible light. One is ultraviolet A (UVA) which is the ray that produces a tan, but is more linked to deadly melanoma and causes skin damage and aging (think wrinkles and "old age" skin spots). The other is ultraviolet B (UVB), which causes the uncomfortable sunburn. This year in the U.S. there will be approximately 76,000 new cases of melanoma with some 9,000 deaths.

The damaging rays from the sun are most intense between the hours of 10 AM and 4 PM.

These are my suggestions:

- Always start the summer season with a new fresh tube of sunscreen; price has nothing to do with performance. Also use a sun screen lip balm.

- Use a sunscreen with an SPF rating of at least 30. Higher than 50 is probably not necessary. SPF literally means "sun protection factor" and measures how well a sunscreen protects your skin.

A sunscreen should be labeled "broad spectrum" protecting against both UVA and UVB, and be water and sweat resistant. There is no commercial sunscreen on the market that is water proof.

- Apply liberally. Use at least 1 ounce (2 tablespoons, enough to fill a shot glass) for your entire body, and apply liberally to the face, ears, and neck.

- Don't overlook applying to feet, back of neck, behind the knees, and bald spots on the scalp..

- Apply at least 20 minutes before sun exposure, every 2 hours thereafter, and immediately after you swim or perspire. Avoid using sunscreen sprays on children as they can inhale the chemical ingredients. Spray it onto your hands and rub it onto their skin or use only the lotion form.

- Whenever possible, wear light colored tight knit clothing and brimmed hats while in the sun.  Wear sunglasses rated to block UVA and UVB rays.

- Avoid tanning salons where damage to the skin can be equal to the damage from the sun.

It should also be noted that the commonly used chemical sun screens have not been proven to be toxic to humans when used as recommended, and that the so called "natural" sunscreens have not proven to be as effective as claimed.

Enjoy your outdoor summer activities, but do yourselves and especially your children a favor, and protect your/their skin from both damage and cancer by properly using a good sunscreen product.

## Difficulty Sleeping

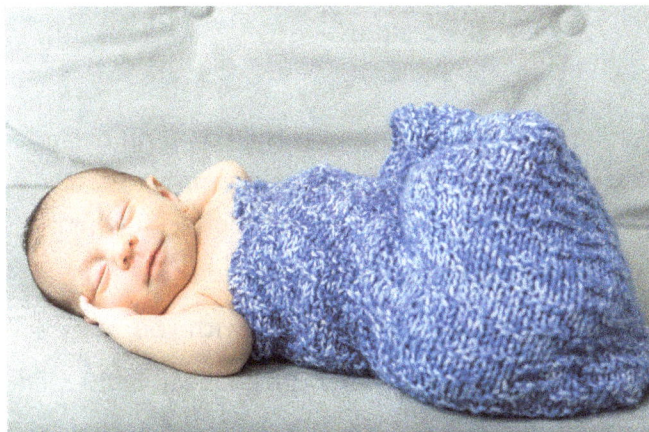

It is estimated that about one third of our population suffers from some form of insomnia. For some, it is severe and chronic, but for others it can be mild. Insomnia can be due to factors such as pain, illness, anxiety, or recent travel. Insomnia can make us feel chronically tired, cranky, and irritable. Left untreated, insomnia is linked to increased illness or morbidity. There is a wealth of research indicating that people with insomnia have poorer overall health, more work absenteeism, and a higher incidence of depression.

Many insomnia sufferers will turn to drugs to help them sleep. Most begin with over the counter medications, which usually contain an antihistamine as the main ingredient. (Men with enlarged prostates should avoid use of antihistamines.) Antihistamines cause drowsiness and may help one to fall asleep. They are relatively safe but can cause a reduced level of alertness the next day. Food supplements and herbal sleep remedies, such as melatonin and valerian, may help but they are unregulated and have unpredictable results.

If your insomnia persists more than a week or two, you may want to consult with your doctor. Before you do, it would be a good idea to keep a sleep log for one week. Here's what you would want to record:

- The time you go to bed, the time you get up, and the approximate amount of time you were awake during the night

263

- Drugs you take, including the use of alcohol, caffeine, and tobacco
- Disturbing factors, such as pain, a new born baby, a snoring bed partner, or noise outside the bedroom
- Whether you feel rested upon arising

Treating insomnia with prescription medication is a common treatment for these sleep problems. These medications for the treatment of insomnia are called hypnotics and need to be prescribed by your doctor. They should only be taken when:

- The cause of your insomnia has been evaluated
- The sleep problems are causing difficulties with your daily activities
- Appropriate sleep promoting behaviors have been addressed

All hypnotics induce sleep and some will help to maintain sleep. They work by acting on areas in the brain believed to be involved in sleep promotion. They are the drugs of choice because they have the highest benefit and the lowest risk as sleep-promoting drugs.

Your health care provider may want to interview your bed partner about the quantity and quality of your sleep. In some cases, you may be referred to a sleep center for special tests.

# Sleep Apnea

Sleep apnea is a common disorder and a potentially deadly condition, in which the airway briefly becomes blocked during sleep, causing one to temporarily stop breathing. These pauses last from seconds to minutes, and can occur up to 5-30 times per hour. Sleep apnea is a common condition affecting some 25 million Americans. It robs one of a good night's sleep, causing excessive daytime drowsiness and feeling constantly tired.

The main types of sleep apnea are:

- Obstructive sleep apnea, the most common form that occurs when throat muscles relax.
- Central sleep apnea, occurs when the brain doesn't send proper signals to the muscles that control breathing.

It's also possible to have both types of sleep apnea at the same time.

Most people who suffer from sleep apnea aren't aware of the condition and may think they are getting a decent sleep. They are frequently tipped off by a family member or bed partner, who is aware of the sufferer's nocturnal breathing difficulties.

Sleep apnea occurs when the muscles in the back of the throat relax, which can temporarily narrow and even close off the airway. The brain then senses the lack of oxygen and awakens one enough to take a normal breath, and so the cycle continues.

Symptoms of sleep apnea are:

- Making loud snoring or choking sounds during sleep
- Loud snoring (not everyone who snores has sleep apnea)
- Excessive daytime sleeping and drowsiness
- Observed episodes of not breathing during sleep

- Awakening with dry mouth or sore throat
- Abrupt awakening feeling short of breath

Common risk factors for sleep apnea are:

- Being obese
- Being male or elderly
- Use of medications such as, sleeping medications and tranquilizers, as well as alcohol and tobacco
- Medical conditions such as hypertension and hypothyroidism

Sleep apnea is diagnosed on the basis of family and medical histories, a physical exam, and from sleep studies done at specialized sleep clinics. These sleep studies monitor you during sleep and can definitively determine if you have sleep apnea and how severe it is.

## Celiac Disease

There is much talk these days about gluten free food and gluten free diets. I'd like to explain what this is all about.

Gluten is a protein found in foods containing wheat, barley, or rye. The consumption of gluten by susceptible individuals causes celiac disease, which affects the digestive system. People with celiac disease who eat gluten containing food experience an immune reaction, which damages the lining of their small intestines. This damage interferes with the intestines ability to absorb certain nutrients, which over time can deprive many of our vital organs of proper nourishment.

The most common symptoms of celiac disease are abdominal pain, vomiting, bloating, and diarrhea. Less common symptoms are depression, irritability, joint pains, upset stomach, cramps, rashes, and weight loss. Infants and young children seem to have more of the digestive symptoms than do adults.

About 3 million people in the U.S. have celiac disease. Having a family member with celiac disease does raise one's risk of the disease.

Diagnosing celiac disease can be difficult because some of its symptoms are similar to other illnesses, such as irritable bowel syndrome, diverticulitis, intestinal infections, and chronic fatigue syndrome. Diagnosis rates are increasing as doctors become more aware of the variety of symptoms of this disease and as reliable blood tests become more available. A biopsy of the small intestine can be done to confirm the diagnosis.

At this time there is no cure for celiac disease but it can be managed by a proper diet. For most people following a gluten free diet will alleviate the symptoms, heal the damaged intestinal lining, and prevent further damage. Once beginning the diet, symptomatic improvement can occur within days, but it may take many months for the small intestine to heal itself. To stay well, one needs to be on a gluten free diet for the remainder of their lives.

In spite of having celiac disease, one can still eat a well-balanced, healthy, and tasty diet. Wheat flour can be substituted by using rice, soy, potato, quinoa, buckwheat, or bean flour. There are now a wide variety of gluten free pastas, breads, snacks, and other foods.

People with celiac disease must be careful about food they buy at school, work, or restaurants, as well as food purchased at grocery stores. Eating out can be a challenge to avoid gluten containing foods.

Here are some examples of common foods and beverages to avoid unless they are labeled gluten free:

- Bread
- Cakes, pies, cookies, crackers, and croutons
- Processed luncheon meats and gravies
- Salad dressings and sauces (including soy sauce)
- Soups
- Beer

Oats are technically free of gluten but are frequently contaminated with it. Be sure the oats label states that it is free of gluten.

See your doctor if you think you are having any symptoms of celiac disease to confirm the diagnosis and work on a treatment plan.

# Constipation

Constipation is not exactly a dinner topic, but it is a condition that affects almost every living person at one time or another. It's a common complaint at the doctor's office.

Constipation is defined as infrequent bowel movements or difficult passage of stools. The normal number of bowel movements for adults ranges from one or more per day to 2-3 per week. For most people going without a bowel movement for several days is a temporary condition and does not lead to any obvious discomfort or health problems. One may begin feeling uncomfortable when constipation lasts more than a few days. It should be noted that constipation does not build up toxins in the gut, nor does it lead to cancer.

There are many causes of constipation, some of the more common being:
- Inadequate amounts of fiber in your diet
- Insufficient liquid intake
- Lack of physical activity
- Side effect of some medications, especially narcotic pain medications, such as Vicoden and Percocet
- Changes in daily routine or lifestyle
- Colon cancer (rare)

There are two approaches for dealing with constipation:

**Lifestyle changes**
- A high fiber diet including beans, whole grains, fresh fruits and vegetables, and less dairy, red meat, and processed foods
- Adequate fluid intake
- Regular exercise
- Trying not to delay a bowel movement when one has the urge

## Laxatives

- Fiber supplements are natural and very safe. Examples include Metamucil and FiberCon, which are safe and effective to use daily.

- Stool softeners, such as Colace and Surfak, add moisture to the stool.

- Stimulants help increase intestinal motility. Examples include Dulcolax, Senekot, and Correctol (best not to use too often).

- Osmotics bring more fluid into the intestines causing easier passage of stool. One of the most common which I recommend is Miralax, available without a prescription.

- Saline laxatives also help to draw fluid into the intestines. Examples include milk of magnesia and Haley's M-O.

- Lubricants, such as a dose of mineral oil, help the intestines to pass the stool more easily.

My personal favorite regimen is to use the osmotic Miralax first, followed within a day or two by a stimulant such as Dulcolax. See your doctor if none of the above products seem to be helping.

I want to take this opportunity to talk about colon cleansing, which is enema therapy claimed to help flush the toxins out of the colon. There is absolutely no scientific proof that there are toxins in the colon that can cause any harm. Most substances, good or bad, have been absorbed into the body in the small intestine, which is not affected by enemas. In fact, colon cleansing can flush out needed electrolytes before they can be absorbed by the colon and also wash out beneficial intestinal bacteria. Don't flush your money down the toilet on this misguided treatment.

# Diverticulitis

Many people these days who are having routine colon screening exams, are being told that they have a condition called diverticulosis, which is the presence of small pockets or pouches in the wall of the large bowel found just above the rectum. Risk factors for diverticulosis include inadequate intake of dietary fiber, lack of exercise, and aging. Diverticula are found in up to 60% of people by age 60, and the percentage keeps climbing with age.

Most people who are told they have this condition are surprised to find this out, because they have had and probably will never have any symptoms of the disease. However, at some point in time, 10% to 20% of those who have diverticula will develop an infection in one of these pouches, which is then called *diverticulitis*. (The suffix "itis" means inflammation.) It has long been thought that eating popcorn, nuts, or seeds would contribute to diverticulitis by becoming trapped in a diverticula, but this has since been disproven.

Common symptoms of diverticulitis are increasing pain and tenderness in the left lower abdomen, fever, nausea, and either diarrhea or constipation. Your doctor will likely order a blood count which may show an increase in the white blood cells indicating an active infection. A CAT scan of the abdomen will often confirm the diagnosis.

Most of those in the early stages of diverticulitis can be treated as an outpatient with antibiotics for up to 2 weeks, pain medicine as needed, and a liquid diet for a few days. In most cases this is all the treatment that is necessary. If there is no significant improvement in 2-3 days, or if symptoms worsen at any time, a prompt medical re-evaluation is necessary.

Potential complications of diverticulitis necessitating immediate hospitalization are:
- An infected diverticula filled with pus (called an abscess)
- Rupture of an infected diverticula spilling contents of the bowel into the abdominal cavity, which can lead to a life threatening infection
- A bowel obstruction, when the bowel is blocked and stops working

At this stage, treatment will include powerful intravenous antibiotics, IV fluids with no liquids or food by mouth, and adequate pain control. Surgery may be needed on an emergency basis to remove the infected bowel, or it may be delayed and done at a later date when the infection/inflammation has calmed down.

Up to 40% of those who have recovered from non-complicated diverticulitis will have one or many more attacks in the future.

If you have worsening pain in the left lower abdomen or no improvement of pain for a few days, whether or not you know you have diverticular disease, seek medical help immediately.

# Food Poisoning

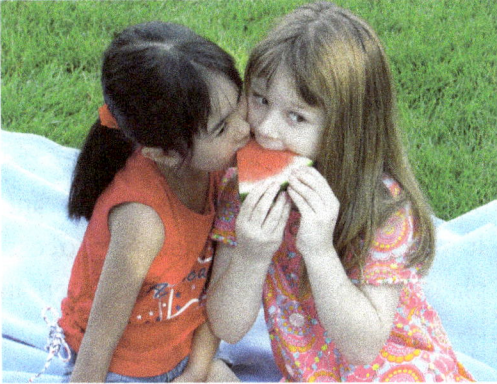

Summer is the time for picnics and social gatherings. This brings about an increased chance of food poisoning, which is vomiting and/or diarrhea that comes about from eating contaminated food. The most common form of food poisoning is from infectious organisms, such as bacteria and viruses. When eating outside the home, these organisms can contaminate food at any point during its production, processing, or serving. More commonly, contamination can also occur in the home. This happens because of food that is improperly handled, incorrectly cooked, or inadequately stored. The most common food culprits are chicken products, fish, and shellfish. Another common source of food poisoning is from food that has been cooked and left unrefrigerated for too long, especially at buffets and outdoor picnics.

Steps to prevent food poisoning:

1.  Wash hands, utensils, and food prep surfaces frequently and thoroughly with soap and water

2.  Keep raw foods separate from ready to eat foods

3.  Cook foods to a safe temperature

4.  Refrigerate or freeze perishable foods promptly

5.  "When in doubt-throw it out"

Signs and symptoms of food poisoning may start within hours or up to one to two days after eating the contaminated food. The most common symptoms of food poisoning are nausea, vomiting, stomach cramps, and diarrhea. The vomiting and diarrhea are the body's way of eliminating the contaminated food.

There is no easy method to differentiate between food poisoning and common stomach flu other than if more than one person comes down with vomiting and/or diarrhea after eating a common meal, then food poisoning is the probable culprit. Fortunately, the symptoms of either food poisoning, or of stomach flu, are usually mild and often resolve without treatment.

The best treatment for food poisoning is to let it run its course.  In most cases, once the body rids itself of the contaminated food, the symptoms improve. For this reason, anti diarrhea medicine is not recommended because it may slow down the healing process. If diarrhea must be controlled because of travel plans or work responsibilities, then an over the counter medication, such as Imodium may be helpful.

 The main goal of treatment is to replace lost body fluids to prevent dehydration. This can be done by drinking lots of liquids, such as electrolyte drinks for adults or Pedialyte for children. A proven method to help prevent dehydration in spite of frequent vomiting, is to take frequent small sips of clear liquids until vomiting stops

When to seek medical attention:
- Inability to keep any liquids down for more than 6-8 hours
- No urine production for 6-8 hours
- Mild vomiting or diarrhea lasting more than 2-3 days
- Blood in vomit or diarrhea
- Fever
- Severe abdominal pain

Have a safe and enjoyable summer. Bon appetit!

# Lactose Intolerance

Most of us have heard of lactose intolerance, which to those who have it, can cause abdominal cramping, bloating, gas, and diarrhea. Symptoms usually begin within 30 minutes to several hours after eating or drinking foods with lactose, also known as milk sugar. This condition can be quite uncomfortable, but harmless. Other conditions causing similar symptoms include irritable bowel syndrome, inflammatory bowel disease, and overuse of laxatives.

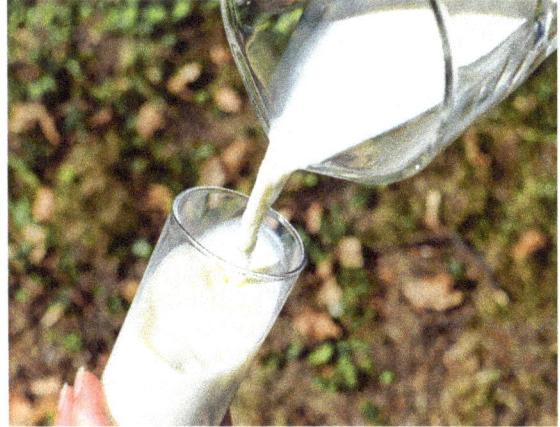

Lactose intolerance is relatively common in adults, occurring more frequently, in Native Americans, and people of Asian, African, and South American descent, than inthose of European descent. Symptoms usually develop during the teen or adult years and become even more common as you get older, with a reported worldwide incidence of 75 percent of adults being lactose intolerant.

Lactose is composed of two simple sugars called glucose and galactose. Lactose intolerance occurs when your own  small intestine does not produce enough of an enzyme called lactase which is needed  to break down lactose into the glucose and galactose. Although these two simple sugars will be absorbed through the intestinal wall into the blood stream, undigested lactose will not. It will simply pass through the gut, where it will interact with normal bacteria causing the signs and symptoms of lactose intolerance.

The best way to determine if you are lactose intolerant is to avoid eating all dairy products and see if the symptoms go away. If they do, then you can begin adding small amounts of them back to your diet and see if the symptoms return.

In reality, there is probably no significant benefit to our health from consuming dairy products past weaning. Since there is no cure for lactose intolerance, your best bet if you want to consume dairy products is to treat your symptoms by avoiding or limiting milk products. If you choose to continue to consume dairy products, saving milk for mealtimes only can help lessen symptoms. You can also use lactose free milk or substitute with soy milk. Over the counter lactase enzyme supplements such as Lact-Aid and Dairy Ease can be taken just before a meal or snack. Cultured yogurt is also fairly well tolerated.

For those who are concerned about consuming enough natural calcium, other non dairy foods contain calcium, including broccoli, kale, calcium fortified cereals and juices, canned fish, and soy products.

If you choose to consume dairy products and are having symptoms that concern you, see your doctor who will help you manage this bothersome but not serious condition.

# Living with Multiple Myeloma

## Dr. Hollenbeck's Personal Journey

It was late on a Friday afternoon in October, 2013, when I received the dreaded phone call from my oncologist telling me that the latest blood tests confirmed I had a type of cancer called *multiple myeloma*. This is a cancer of the plasma cells, which are found in the blood and produce antibodies for our immune system. These malignant cells multiply rapidly and can cause damage throughout the body, especially affecting bones and kidneys, ultimately leading to death within two years if left untreated. What shocking and life-changing news that was! I don't believe that anyone can fully feel the impact of such news unless one has experienced it oneself.

For me, it was an end to life as usual. I seemed to be sailing along quite well, having survived **68** years with only minimal health problems. I was still working full-time (with no intention of retiring), exercising regularly on my bicycle, following my own advice on keeping up with routine health maintenance, not smoking since a few wayward years in my youth, drinking alcohol responsibly, and just taking good care of myself. Life seemed to be humming along quite well, until I heard that dreaded *cancer* word.

My first thought was, am I going to die soon or at least begin to suffer as the cancer would progress? What is going to happen to my wife Beth and daughter Emma without me around? Will they be able to take care of themselves, the house, and the finances? Was I going to be able to keep working? How drastically is our life going to change? What is going to happen to me now?

After Beth and I had a good cry together, I spent that weekend researching my diagnosis. I was somewhat encouraged that medical science had gotten to the point where, although the disease is still considered "incurable" and "terminal," it is at least considered treatable, with survival rates for most patients with myeloma measured in years, and for some fortunate people even a few decades. Some of the studies go so far as to say that a cure (a term rarely used in cancer these days) is in the not too distant future – hopefully soon enough to cure my disease.

As I explain in the cancer section of this book, multiple myeloma involves the antibody-producing plasma cells found in the bone marrow. Myeloma's effect on bone causes extreme osteoporosis (thinning of bones), which brought about my first symptom of back pain. This was due to several of the vertebral bones of my spine collapsing, which is referred to as *compression fractures*. Blood tests were done to find out why an otherwise healthy guy like me would have these fractures. The specific test for myeloma was positive. The next step was a bone marrow biopsy to determine the severity of the disease. This procedure involved numbing the skin over the back of my pelvic bone and inserting a needle into the bone marrow to obtain a specimen for more detailed evaluation.

I then began a two-month course of chemotherapy at our oncology infusion center here in Santa Cruz. I received three drugs. One was given as a shot (not by IV), and the other two were in pill form. One of the pills costs $700 per pill! I learned this is not an uncommon price for the new generation of cancer drugs. My particular course of chemotherapy did not cause me to lose my hair, make me sick to my stomach, or any other of the common chemotherapy side effects. I was feeling pretty smug about how I was sailing through the therapy when finally a side effect caught up with me. I developed numbness of my feet and my hands, a condition called *peripheral neuropathy*. It continues to cause me some difficulty walking and maintaining my balance.

In order to treat the ongoing back pain from my compression fractures, I had a procedure called *kyphoplasty* done by a spine surgeon at UCSF (The University of California San Francisco). This procedure involved my receiving general anesthesia, followed by the surgeon inserting a large needle into each of four compressed vertebral bones. Through the needle, a small balloon is blown up to help open up the collapsed bone. The balloon is then removed and a rapid-drying cement-like substance is injected into the boney space. This helps to restore some integrity to the compressed bone and keeps it from collapsing further. It also usually improves the associated back pain, which fortunately proved true for me.

As the course of my treatment continued, the scheduled stem cell transplant that I was to receive at UCSF was postponed because of the neuropathy, and treatment was put on hold, until tests showed that the cancer had relapsed. After leaving work again and beginning a new round of chemotherapy, I decided to officially retire after 43 years of medical practice. It was time to take care of myself, plus I felt that my neuropathy and significant decreased energy level prevented me from providing the highest quality care to patients.

It has been five years now since I received the diagnosis and undertook treatment. In general, I feel well and am learning to live with the neuropathy of my feet, as disabling as it has become. I try to push myself by exercising as much as I am able to do, which I think is helping me feel better. I would recommend exercise, to the best of one's ability, to anyone suffering a chronic disease as part of an overall treatment program.

I've never allowed myself to indulge in a pity party over my cancer diagnosis, nor do I blame God, myself, or any other possible causative factors. It is what it is. I trust in God and the medical system in which I trained and practiced to do the best to treat my cancer and maintain my quality of life. My job now is to take good care of myself, enjoy quality time with family and friends, and continue living as normal a life as possible.

# Dr. Hollenbeck's Biography

I was born into a family of doctors in Milwaukee, Wisconsin, so it was natural for me to follow in their footsteps. Making house calls (yes, there was such a thing back then) and hospital rounds with my father was exciting to me. After graduating from The Medical College of Wisconsin in 1971, I came to California to do an internship at the Santa Clara Valley Medical Center in San Jose with the intention of returning to practice medicine in Milwaukee, but California grabbed a hold of me and never let go.

I stayed at "The Valley," as we called it, and worked in the outpatient clinic and became chief jail physician for the Santa Clara County Jail as well as the Elmwood Correctional Facility. During this time I thoroughly enjoyed moonlighting in the emergency room at The Valley. At the end of 1974, I was approached by a group of physicians who were taking over the emergency room contracts at the Valley Medical Center and at San Jose Hospital, to join with them for full-time emergency medical work. I worked in emergency medicine for the next five years. It was very challenging and exciting and provided me great experience in practicing emergency care as well as providing routine medical care.

It was also a time when I accepted Christ as my personal savior. With this new change came a desire to do medical mission work, and through the Christian Medical Society, I was assigned to work in the Central American country of Honduras. I spent two years there on the Miskito Coast on the Caribbean side of the country, the first year with Dr. Sam Marx at his well-established clinic, then the second year moving to a small coastal town called Cocobila. There I helped to establish a clinic and train several women to function as nurses to care for the local Miskito Indian population.

I joined the Santa Cruz Medical Clinic in 1987 when it opened its first satellite office in Scotts Valley and spent 28 wonderful years practicing urgent care medicine. I came to know many wonderful people in the community during that time, having had around 100,000 patient visits.

I retired at the end of 2015, and I am enjoying retirement. I can now spend more time with my wife, Beth, who is very busy as a music educator. She also keeps me busy by involving me in her community activism.

I have three children, Emma, Blake, and Brandon. Emma and Blake are attending college and enjoy working in local restaurants.

I've thoroughly enjoyed working with our local community, and it's been a true pleasure for me to give back to it through my articles in the Press-Banner. I began writing them more than ten years ago and have had some 200 articles published to date. My mission in writing the articles was to share my years of experience in a format that was easily understandable and informative, and to help promote better health within our community.

# Index

*Note: Pages in bold refer to full article*

www.ingramcontent.com/pod-product-compliance
Lightning Source LLC
Chambersburg PA
CBHW080231270326
41926CB00020B/4202